DISEASES IN HISTORY
Malaria

Diseases in History

Malaria

Kevin Cunningham

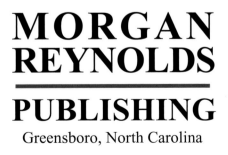

MORGAN REYNOLDS

PUBLISHING

Greensboro, North Carolina

Diseases in History

PLAGUE

FLU

MALARIA

HIV/AIDS

DISEASES IN HISTORY: MALARIA

Copyright © 2009 By Kevin Cunningham

Library of Congress Cataloging-in-Publication Data

Cunningham, Kevin, 1966-
  Diseases in history. Malaria / by Kevin Cunningham.
     p. cm.
  Includes bibliographical references and index.
  ISBN-13: 978-1-59935-103-2
  ISBN-10: 1-59935-103-X
  1. Malaria--History. I. Title. II. Title: Malaria.
  RC160.C86 2009
  614.5'32--dc22

                                             2008051619

Printed in the United States of America
First Edition

Contents

Introduction..10

Chapter One
    The Adversaries 14

Chapter Two
    The Roman Disease 22

Chapter Three
    The Fever Tree and the Magic Bullet 41

Chapter Four
    Eradication..72

Chapter Five
    Disease of the Poor 97

Sources..122
Bibliography..126
Web sites 138
Glossary 140
Index 143

Introduction

The world's most dangerous malaria lurks along Thailand's borders. There, the parasites that cause the disease can resist all the established drugs. Southeast Asia has bred super-malaria strains for a long time. Forty-some years ago the local malaria evolved until it overcame chloroquine, the miracle drug that was supposed to destroy the disease for good. People with the resistant parasites in their bodies then returned to their homes in nations across Asia, or to jobs in Africa. Now, the malaria in those places resists the old drugs, too.

All the factors that contribute to malaria are present in Southeast Asia. There is a wet and humid climate loved by the mosquitoes that carry the disease. There is environmental change. As logging cuts into the rain forest, the shock to the ecological system means that only those species that thrive in changing landscapes—like mosquitoes—can adjust. Mining along the Cambodian border tears up the environment further. The fortune hunters there hope to fend off malaria just long enough to cash in and get out.

There is poverty. More than 400,000 refugees from Myanmar live in Thailand. They have fled the civil war in their own country and live in camps. The refugees face the hardships common to displaced people everywhere—poor housing and sanitation, inadequate food and medicine, and an environment overstrained by hundreds of thousands of desperate human beings.

Malaria takes advantage of human problems just as it does humanity's habit of altering the environment. The refugees get ill from the disease, as do the miners and the soldiers, the aid workers, and the scientists.

Centuries ago, Italians gave the malady the name *mal'aria*—mal meaning bad, aria meaning air. They shared the widespread belief that the swamps nearby coughed up unhealthy "airs" that caused disease. To the English the disease was the ague, to the French *la paludisme*, to the ancients swamp fever in many languages. People in one part of Mali call it by a word that means "sickness of the green season" because it arrives with the rains.

Malaria has caused human suffering since prehistory. A form of it afflicted the prehuman ancestors of *Homo sapiens* before that. Since then, malaria has killed more human beings than any other disease. There are historians who say it has killed half the people who have ever lived.

Human beings have constantly tried out new strategies and tools against it. Some tribes of Vietnamese hill people, recognizing that the local mosquitoes fly low, keep their sleeping platforms ten feet off the ground. Ancient Roman philosophers, though unaware insects carried malaria, recognized the disease had a connection to buggy swamps and warned people not to buy property near such places. Shepherds in many lands learned to get their animals to higher, cooler ground before evening came and the mosquitoes fed.

Every culture encountering the disease came up with a variety of advice, medicines, and magic spells. The English boiled bark from the white willow (*Salix alba*), a tree that grew in marshy areas. Nigeria's Hausa people used thirty or more plants for fevers, and the peoples of Madagascar many more. Ancient Romans made offerings to Febris, goddess of fevers.

"There is no aspect of life in [a malarial] country which is not affected, either directly or indirectly, by this disease," said malariologist J. A. Sinton in 1936. "It constitutes one of the most important causes of economic misfortune, engendering poverty, diminishing the quantity and quality of the food supply, lowering the physical and intellectual standard of the nation, and hampering increased prosperity and economic progress in every way."

Today malaria is considered a disease of the poor, and Sinton's words apply wherever it remains severe. But the disease has never respected the powerful, either. It may have killed Alexander the Great and Genghis Khan. Julius Caesar suffered, as Shakespeare knew when he wrote, "He had a fever when he was in Spain, and when the fit was on him, I did mark how he did shake." The list of other famous victims includes the poet Byron and the painter Caravaggio, the writers Laura Ingalls Wilder and Arthur Conan Doyle, and a fair number of the legendary explorers that dared the New World's rivers or the unmapped African interior.

Defying modern medicine as it once defied Febris, malaria has surged back. Between 300 and 500 million people suffer its symptoms every year. Many years, 2 to 3 million of them die. Most are pregnant African women and African children under the age of five.

The spread of malaria today is the latest period of a contest that has gone on for thousands of years. When it comes to malaria, humanity's adversaries are persistent and quick to change. Yet at first glance they seem too inconsequential to cause the harm they do. After all, one is a tiny parasite that can't be seen without a microscope. The other is the mosquito.

A close-up photograph of an *Anopheles minimus* mosquito, a species that carries malaria, feeding on a human host. *(Courtesy of Geoff du Feu/Alamy)*

one
The
Adversaries

Mosquitoes predate humans by millions of years. We know because specimens very much like those that annoy us today have been found suspended in amber that coagulated eons ago. Today, there are approximately 3,500 known species. Hundreds more species, perhaps thousands, have yet to be catalogued by humans.

Their breathtaking ability to adapt allows them to live in almost every surface habitat on Earth. For example, breeding grounds can include swamps, irrigation pools, and even old tires on container ships. Their range covers the high latitudes to the equator. In the Arctic, a swarm can suck dry an entire caribou. In the African desert, the eggs of one species are laid already infected with disease and remain dormant until rains come, even if it takes years.

Different species even attack people in different ways. *Aedes aegypti*, the carrier of yellow fever, likes to bite human ankles, while *Ochlerotatus sollicitans*, the New Jersey mosquito, strikes from above.

A disease-carrying animal is called a *vector*. All malaria-carrying mosquitoes, or malaria vectors, belong to the genus *Anopheles*. There are more than four hundred *Anopheles* species. As with all mosquitoes, only *Anopheles* females need blood because the females carry the eggs. The smaller and shyer males prefer plant nectar or other foods.

When the time comes, the female *Anopheles* zeroes in on a blood source. A number of factors guide the insect, including body heat, moisture, and the carbon dioxide we exhale. Recent research suggests the mosquitoes that bite humans may key on certain odors. Smelly human feet seems to be a favorite for some.

Once settled on the skin, the mosquito tests with its proboscis until it finds blood. A chemical in its saliva blocks blood coagulation in the victim.

An *Anopheles* mosquito feeds in a distinctive pose, with its rear end in the air. Ninety seconds or so after the meal, having taken in blood equal to two or three times its body weight (and possibly having passed on malaria), the female flies away and lands on the first vertical surface it can find. There the insect's system separates water from the blood. It urinates the water. The eggs inside its body feed on the blood.

The eggs are soon laid in whatever type of water the species prefers. Once the larvae hatch, predators start prowling for a meal. Fish eat mosquito larvae, as does *Toxorhynchites*, the world's largest mosquito. Other threats abound—excessive heat or cold, insufficient food, and the evaporation of the water can kill larvae. Those that survive mature into mosquitoes and fly off to feed and mate.

Mosquitoes only carry malaria. The disease's direct cause is a microscopic parasite that uses the insect to hatch its eggs and inject its offspring into animals.

The parasite belongs to the genus *Plasmodium*. Four *Plasmodium* species cause malaria in human beings. Twenty or so more do the same to monkeys and apes, with still others infecting lizards, their distant cousins the birds, and other animals.

Millennia of contact with us have turned the four human malaria parasites into highly specialized organisms. To grow, these *Plasmodia* require our liver cells, to feed they need our red blood cells. While humans don't need the parasites, the parasites need us.

The malaria *Plasmodium* starts out as a thread-shaped sporozoite bursting from a pouch on the stomach wall of a female mosquito. From there the sporozoites make their way to the insect's saliva glands. There they wait until the female feeds. As the insect draws up blood for its eggs, the sporozoites migrate the other way into the human bloodstream.

Once in the body, the sporozoites move into the liver and begin a complex series of transformations inside liver cells. There each sporozoite reproduces itself thousands of times. The human host, meanwhile, feels fine.

After anywhere from six to seventeen days, the expanded population of sporozoites pours out of the liver and floods the bloodstream. Each one clamps onto a red blood cell and devours the hemoglobin inside. The victim's body temperature soars, sometimes to as high as 106 degrees Fahrenheit. A headache pounds the skull. After hours of fever the chills set in. Papua New Guineans call the chills the *guria*—the earthquake—and it's an accurate description. Finally, the victim breaks into a sweat that soaks clothes and bed sheets.

The cycle then repeats. Subsequent malaria attacks come in waves, with peaks every thirty-six, forty-eight, or seventy-two hours (depending on the type of parasite). The cycles continue until (1) the body's immune system fights off the parasites; (2) the victim takes anti-malaria drugs; or (3) death.

Though the severity of the symptoms suggests the parasites overwhelm the body's defenses, a healthy human immune system actually destroys around 90 percent of the parasitic attackers.

An illustration of the life cycle of the *Plasmodium* parasites that cause malaria. *(Courtesy of Centers for Disease Control and Prevention)*

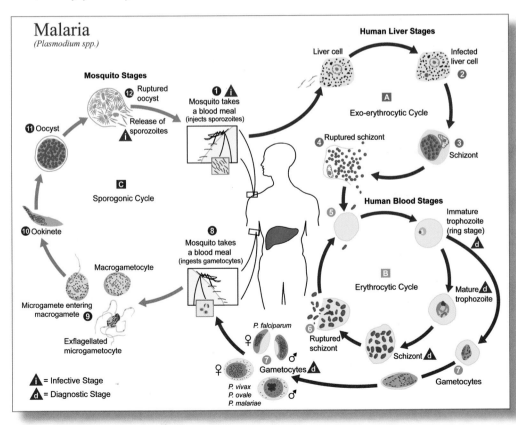

A so-called mild case can also bring on vomiting and muscle aches. Severe cases enlarge the spleen and can cause the liver or kidneys to fail. Anemia (loss of red blood cells) and dehydration are constant risks. The deadliest form of malaria clogs blood pathways to the brain and can cause permanent neurological damage and death. Without medicine, the disease can linger in the body for months or years, and explode into a new attack without warning.

The union of mosquito and parasite—persistent pest and creature invisible to the naked eye—succeeded in spreading malaria across much of the human-inhabited world. But humans have also contributed to the success of the disease. Though malaria struck our prehistoric ancestors, it truly became a part of the human experience when *Homo sapiens* gave up the perils of hunting and gathering, and turned to agriculture.

Lethal Consequences

Of the four species that attack humans, *Plasmodium vivax* is most widespread. *Vivax* was often (though not always) the parasite that troubled the United States and northern Europe into the early twentieth century. Attacks last up to six hours. In between, the victim may feel well enough to function, at least until worn out by the shaking and sweating. But a case can last two months, severe ones longer.

Adding to the problem is the fact that *vivax* parasites remain in the liver for up to three years—some sources say five. A victim is vulnerable to an attack as long as he or she hosts the parasite. Long-term exposure can cause many health problems. The spleen may become enlarged. Jaundice damages the liver. Anemia drains energy and threatens both the heart and nervous system. Other effects include depression and infertility. The body, slowly drained of health, becomes vulnerable to all kinds of illness, including new malaria attacks.

Whereas *vivax* slowly weakens victims, *Plasmodium falciparum* is explosively lethal. Today, *falciparum* accounts for 95 percent of all malaria deaths.

Falciparum incubates in the liver more quickly than *vivax* and releases a greater number of parasites into the bloodstream. Whereas *vivax* attacks only young red blood cells, *falciparum* hits cells regardless of age. Often a blood transfusion is needed to head off the fatal anemia caused by massive loss of the cells. At the same time, infected and dead cells cling to the lining of blood vessels, clogging blood pathways. Soon blood cannot flow to the brain. This brings on cerebral malaria. Victims become disoriented. If not treated, they fall into a coma. Death or permanent neurological damage often follows.

Two less common forms of malaria also exist. *Plasmodium malariae* strikes every seventy-two hours. It does not linger in the liver like *vivax*, but instead circulates in the body for many years as a weak infection. The rare *Plasmodium ovale*, found mostly in West Africa, acts a lot like *vivax*, but with longer attacks.

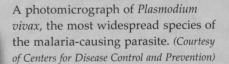

A photomicrograph of *Plasmodium vivax*, the most widespread species of the malaria-causing parasite. *(Courtesy of Centers for Disease Control and Prevention)*

A young boy waits his turn to be tested for malaria in Mozambique, Africa. Most sub-Saharan African countries don't have the medical resources necessary for effective prevention or treatment of malaria. *(Courtesy of AP Images/ Karel Prinsloo)*

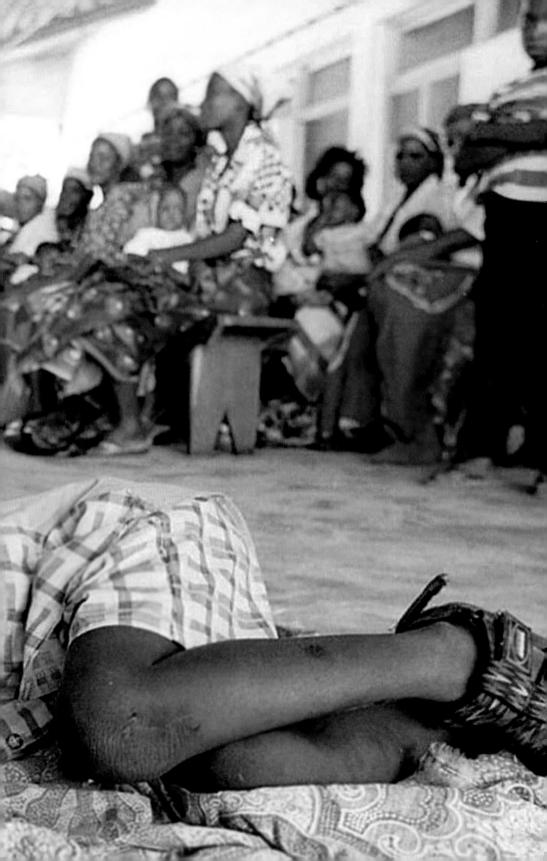

two

The Roman Disease

Slash-and-burn agriculture is as old as, well, agriculture. The earliest farmers practiced it on ancient forests just as modern-day Brazilians do in the Amazonian jungle.

Early farmers, needing land, cut down the vegetation in the fertile rain forest. Over the next few weeks or months the dead vegetation dried. At the same time, the farmers stripped the trees of their bark and left them to die. The next step was to burn the vegetation, both to get it out of the way and cycle a share of its nutrients into the soil underneath. Crops then were sewn, grown, and eaten. Over the next few years the constant planting exhausted the soil nutrients. When that happened, the farmers moved on to a new section of the forest.

While the humans cleared the dense foliage, *Anopheles* mosquitoes discovered farmers. Not long after, the farmers discovered malaria. The insects carried at least three of the malaria parasites—*vivax*, *malariae*, and *ovale*—from other primates to human beings. At some point, enough people became infected to establish malaria in the human population. It's been with people ever since.

Farming provided a more reliable food supply than hunting or gathering. The better-fed, healthier humans had more children. Eventually, people gathered in towns, then cities. Trade and technology followed close behind.

But clearing land for agriculture, like digging mines to get at iron or tin, altered the landscape in dramatic ways. Farming and mining had a way of leaving holes. Holes filled with water gave mosquitoes a place to lay eggs. The insects thrived in environments changed by humans, even as human activity drove other organisms into safer regions (or extinction).

Our records of ancient and pre-ancient times are scanty, so we have no way of knowing when malaria escaped Africa and made its way to Europe and Asia. But existing sources suggest that ancient civilizations recognized the disease. Written descriptions of a malaria-like fever in India date back more than 3000 years. The author of the *Charaka Samhita*, an ancient text on internal medicine, mentioned fevers very much like the forms of malaria.

The ancient Chinese believed that disharmony between yin and yang caused malaria. Fevers with enlarged spleen are mentioned in the *Nei Ching*, a medical text dating from around 2700 BCE. Victims were advised to use certain medicinal plants. According to writers of the time, China's southern region was thick with fevers and other diseases. Wrote Ssu ma Chi'en, "In the area south of the Yangtse the land is low and the climate humid; adult males die young." A man journeying there would, if he was wise, find his wife a new husband before leaving home.

Our firmest evidence of ancient malaria comes from the Greeks. The Greeks didn't understand parasites, but observation made it clear the terrible fevers were related to natural conditions. The group of physician-philosophers writing under the name Hippocrates advised Greeks to avoid marshy waters. Furthermore, Hippocrates said, physicians should consider the season of the year, local water supplies, and living habits when making a diagnosis. "[F]or whenever the great heat comes on suddenly while the earth is soaked by reason of the spring rains . . . the fevers that attack are of the acutest type."

The Greeks recognized the different kinds of malaria. "The least dangerous of all and the mildest and most protracted, is the quartan," Hippocrates said. "What is called semi-tertian . . . is the most fatal." We now know that "quartan"—caused by *P. malariae*—is relatively mild and that "semi-tertian"—caused by *P. falciparum*—is the deadliest.

Hippocrates hypothesized that some agent was responsible. The Greeks blamed *miasma*, a foul-smelling substance they thought was emitted by swamps and marshes. Anyone who has been in a swamp in warm weather can attest to the odor, and the Greeks, like many premodern cultures, related bad smells to sickness. That swamp fever thrived in marshy regions underscored their belief.

Athens, Greece's greatest city, built an empire and dominated the Mediterranean in the fifth century BCE. Malaria was by then endemic in Greece—that is, present in the country at all times. Many historians believe that long-term exposure to debilitating malarial fevers drained the Greeks' energy and good health and contributed to the empire's decline. Greek sources frequently blamed misfortunes and bad decisions on melancholy, a condition we usually call depression—one of malaria's long-term effects.

It's logical to assume that sick and weary workers, both free men and slaves, found it harder to harvest, mine, work metal, sail ships, or fight wars. Population also fell. Malaria struck hard at first-time mothers, affecting fertility, while young children suffered particular harm from *falciparum.*

Weariness and nagging illness, infertility, and depression make it hard for a society to function well. Athens, though still the mightiest empire in the Mediterranean, was already weakened when the Athenians laid siege to Syracuse, the leading city on the island of Sicily. Malaria helped turn what was supposed to be a quick and triumphant war into a disaster that ended Athens' golden age.

Military setbacks forced the Athenians to camp near the marshes west of Syracuse. It would have been hard to think of a worse location, particularly during Sicily's intense summer heat. The stench of marsh, garbage, and excrement hung everywhere. Swarms of disease-bearing mosquitoes, to say nothing of the biting flies, tortured the Athenian soldiers. Their army pinned down, their navy destroyed, the Athenians' strength frittered away, never to be recovered.

A few generations later, the Macedonians to the north swept in and conquered most of Greece. What the Macedonian king Philip started, his son Alexander the Great finished, and expanded into a new empire that stretched from Egypt to the frontier of India.

Alexander returned from India to the city of Babylon, located near modern-day Baghdad. After a boating expedition through the Euphrates River swamps, Alexander came

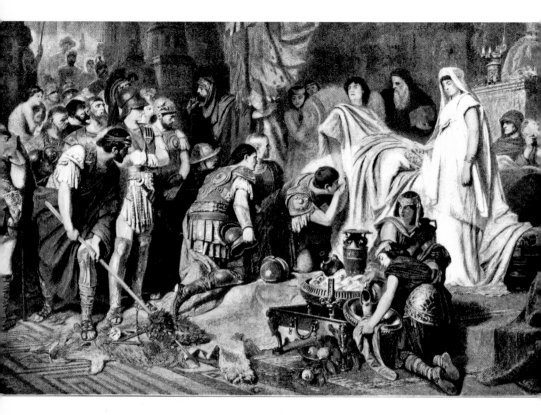

In this nineteenth-century illustration, soldiers pay tribute to a dying Alexander the Great. It is believed that Alexander may have died after contracting malaria while boating through the Euphrates River swamps. *(Courtesy of North Wind Picture Archives/Alamy)*

down with a sudden illness. Whether it was malaria remains in dispute. For a few days Alexander maintained his regular schedule, but soon he was in the grip of raging thirst and a cycle of fever and chills. Eventually paralysis set in—possibly a sign of *falciparum* malaria—and he died.

Like the Greeks, the ancient Romans were wary of marshes. "Precautions should . . . be taken in the neighborhood of swamps," wrote the scholar Varro, "because there are bred

certain minute creatures which cannot be seen by the eyes."
He warned that particular caution had to be exercised when
it came to property near swampland:

"What can I do," asked Fundianus, "to prevent disease if
I should inherit a farm of that kind?"

"Even I can answer that question," replied Agrius, "sell it
for the highest cash price, or if you can't sell it, abandon it."

The Roman version of swamp fever did not spare the high
or low. The emperors Tiberius and Hadrian suffered; fever
struck the young Julius Caesar while he was on the run from
political enemies. Romans built a temple to Febris, the goddess of fever, on Palatine Hill.

The Roman army recognized the goddess's power to ruin
its military adventures. Commanders on the march wisely
considered foul water to be deadly. So did Rome's many enemies. More than once Germanic tribes forced Roman legion-
naires to camp in swamps and damp woods, and waited for
fever to thin their ranks before attacking.

Rome relied on a sophisticated water system to supply the
city and irrigate crops. The system also drained the marshland, particularly in the Campagna, the rich farming region
east of the city. On occasion, however, government oversight
became lax, or manpower or money shortages undercut main-
tenance. Whenever the drainage system fell into disrepair, the
Campagna reverted to its natural marshy state. The mosquitoes soon returned and once again desperate Romans scrib-
bled the magic word *abracadabra* to ward off malaria.

People of the time fought the disease with numerous remedies. In the Near East clarified butter was prescribed. Nearer
to Rome, the physician Galen advised bleeding patients with
malarial fevers (and with most other ailments, for that matter).

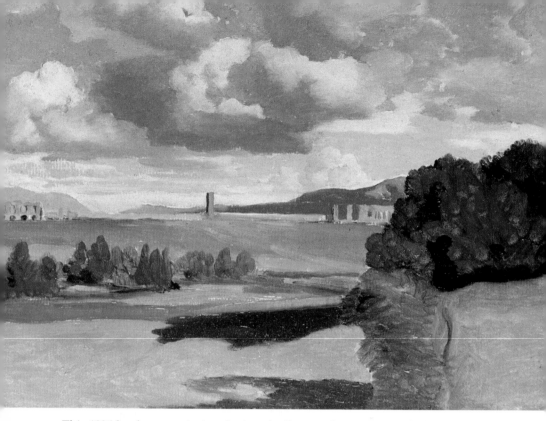

This 1826 landscape painting depicts the Roman Campagna with the ruins of an ancient aqueduct in the distance. In order to remove malarial swamps, Romans utilized a sophisticated water system to drain wetland areas such as the Campagna. *(Courtesy of The Print Collector/Alamy)*

Removing hot blood, he said, cooled the body. Small children who died of malaria were weighed down in their burial receptacles, in hopes of keeping the spirits that brought fever from getting out and harming others.

As Roman society declined, the water and drainage systems began to deteriorate. Agricultural areas reclaimed from marshland reverted to swamp. This reduced harvests and the amount of available food. To work the land the Romans brought in more slaves. Slave labor tended to produce less than free workers. Slaves also revolted, adding violence, disorder, and lost crops to the empire's list of escalating problems.

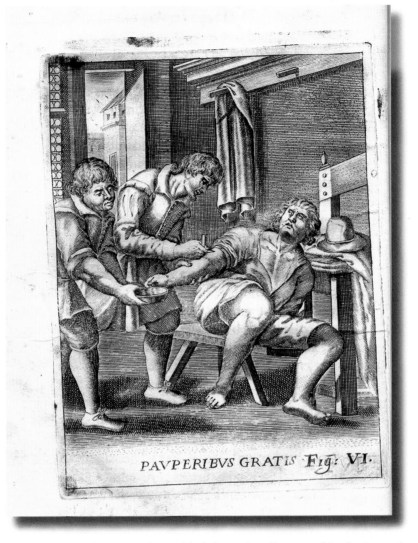

PAVPERIBVS GRATIS Fig: VI.

A 1671 illustration of a patient being bled. In ancient Rome and in the centuries that followed, bleeding was a common treatment for many ailments, including malaria. *(Courtesy of National Library of Medicine)*

By the 400s, Rome was so weak that its citizens relied on epidemics rather than armies to destroy invaders. It worked until Alaric, king of the Visigoths, took and looted Rome in 410. Alaric nonetheless succumbed to a fever soon after, while marching to attack Sicily.

Forty years later another invader, Attila, vowed to take Rome. With a clear path before him, the fearsome king of the Huns suddenly and unexpectedly turned back. According to tradition, Attila had halted to the north of Rome when Pope Leo I arrived with a delegation. Either Leo convinced Attila to break off the invasion, or Attila did so on his own because the Hun army was being hit by an epidemic. Perhaps it was both.

The nature of the epidemic has remained a mystery ever since. Recent archaeological findings suggest a malaria outbreak may have brought about Attila's change in strategy.

Archaeologist David Soren of the University of Arizona excavated a children's cemetery in Lugnano, a town north of Rome. There he found a number of children buried within a short time of one another. The graves also contained sacrificial offerings. He interpreted the discoveries to mean an epidemic caused the locals to despair of help from the Christian god and return to their traditional pagan beliefs to halt the plague.

Signs pointed to malaria. Burnt honeysuckle was one of the offerings—and Romans treated fevers with honeysuckle. Furthermore, the buried children were three years old or younger, the age group most at risk from *falciparum*.

Unlike many diseases, however, malaria leaves only subtle signs on bones, and then only on certain bones. Only in the late 1990s, when DNA testing had advanced enough to allow accurate testing, did researchers confirm that one of the children died of malaria.

Soren dated the cemetery to roughly 450 CE. That places it close to the year—452 CE —the Huns were marauding through Italy. Perhaps Attila learned a lesson from Alaric. He never captured Rome, but he didn't die of malaria, either.

A 1358 illustration of Attila meeting with Pope Leo I outside of Rome. Although it is believed Pope Leo I's plea for mercy convinced Attila to refrain from sacking Rome, archaeological findings suggest a malaria outbreak may have prevented Attila from entering the city.

Even in decline, Rome remained the center of Europe's spiritual world. But being the seat of the western branch of the Catholic Church failed to save it from malaria. The disease struck down so many visiting pilgrims that Europeans referred to it for centuries as the Roman fever or Roman disease. Nor were popes spared. The foreign-born German and French popes who came to dominate the papacy died the same as the pilgrims. Many cardinals, fearing the unhealthy atmosphere, refused to serve in the Holy City.

Malaria spread from the warm Mediterranean to Europe's midlatitudes during the Middle Ages. It was an era when Europeans were clearing the ancient forests to grow more crops. Mosquitoes took advantage. In time it moved as far north as Holland and England. The English called the sickness the *ague*. Shakespeare mentioned it in a dozen works. In fact, many of the London theater-goers watching his plays suffered or had suffered from it. Malarial swamps surrounded where the Houses of Parliament and Big Ben stand today.

Starting in the Middle Ages, and continuing into modern times, epidemics of all kinds brought terror to Europeans. The average person accepted that God sent sickness to punish the world for its sins. There seemed to be no end to His unhappiness. Visitations of bubonic plague appeared out of nowhere. The so-called English sweats, a disease no one had ever seen before, spread death throughout the 1400s. A lethal form of syphilis, possibly imported from the New World, terrorized Europe from the 1490s onward. Tuberculosis spread and great influenza epidemics took place.

Physicians were all but helpless. The medical knowledge of the time could not conceive of parasites or viruses. Whenever an epidemic struck, physicians dug out their leeches to bleed patients while clergymen blamed their sinful congregants for incurring the Almighty's displeasure.

Ordinary people tried to understand disease through a combination of prayer, folk treatments, magic, and superstition. The more religious-minded thought victims babbling with fever were possessed by demons. Beware, one sixteenth-century Italian wrote, of the "numerous illness that night air is wont to generate in human bodies." Malaria, it was believed, might be foiled by shouting a chant up the chimney:

> Tremble and go!
> First day, shiver and burn,
> Tremble and quake!
> Second day, shiver and learn,
> Tremble and die!
> Third day, never return.

Malaria victims learned to cope with lost working days and dying children, with constant weariness and gloom. Only three centuries later, as agriculture became modern—when the forests were long gone and farmers had drained the marshes—did malaria let go of northern Europe.

Meanwhile, the disease found its way to a new, more vulnerable killing ground: the New World.

Colonists arrived on the island of Hispaniola with Columbus's second expedition. European diseases and exploitation decimated the original inhabitants from the first day. Estimates about Hispaniola's pre-Columbian population are controversial, but one figure puts it at about 5 million people. (Others say up to 8 million, still others say much less). Whatever the case, only about 25,000 were left in 1510, less

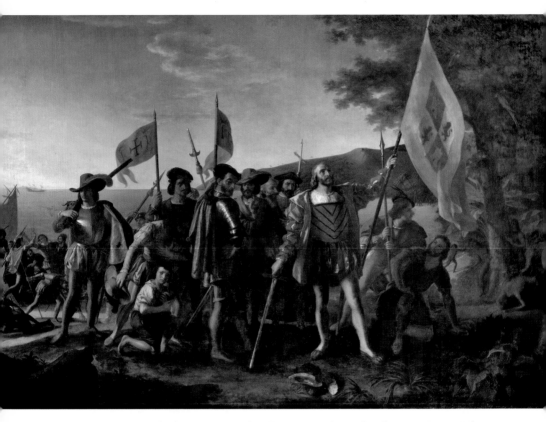

An illustration of Christopher Columbus's expedition landing at Hispaniola in 1492. After Columbus's arrival, the native population was soon decimated by a multitude of European diseases, including malaria. *(Courtesy of Architect of the Capitol)*

than twenty years after Columbus's arrival. Virtually none survived past 1535.

Vivax malaria could have been introduced to the New World by Spanish colonists in the Caribbean, and, separately, the Portuguese in Brazil. The deadlier *falciparum*, however, most likely arrived with African slaves.

Spanish landowners were desperate for laborers for their new mines and plantations. At first they enslaved Hispaniola's surviving natives and abducted tribesmen from the Bahamas and Cuba. But all died too fast to make good slaves. On January 22, 1510, King Ferdinand opened a grim period in history when he agreed to send fifty slaves from Spain. Possibly they were captured Muslims or Canary Islanders; but probably they were Africans in bondage in Spain.

The labor situation worsened after the Spaniards introduced smallpox in 1518. As the native population died out from this horrific new plague, demand for slaves grew. The king sold licenses to slave traders that allowed them to import *bozales*, slaves taken straight from Africa. At some point, *Plasmodium falciparum* carried by *bozales* arrived on one of the early slave ships.

It soon became apparent Africans resisted malaria far more effectively than Europeans. If slaves showed signs of

A 1738 engraving of slaves working at a sugar refinery on a Caribbean island. Desperate for laborers to work in their mines and sugar plantations in the Caribbean, Spanish landowners captured and imported African slaves, who were valued as laborers because of their resistance to malaria. *(Courtesy of The London Art Archive/Alamy)*

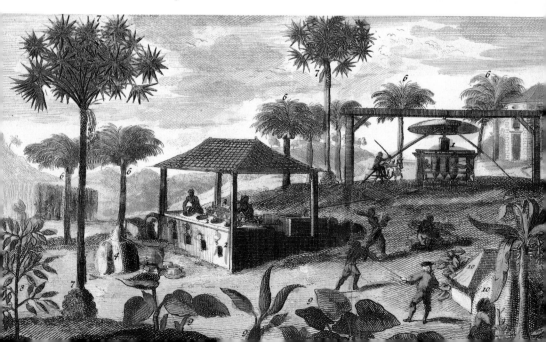

the disease at all it was in a mild version quite unlike the fever that mowed down whites. Malaria thus became part of the lore Europeans believed, and used, to explain their superiority to Africans.

From the earliest days of the slave trade the Spanish had tried to justify the inhuman treatment implicit in slavery. To do so, they used Christian terms. Europeans considered Africans the children of Ham—in Scripture, a race of people condemned to serve others. Racism took this one step further and labeled the Africans as, at best, subhuman. To Europeans, malaria proved this belief was true. That Africans resisted the disease showed that they could not catch the "human" fevers that struck down white Europeans. Similar theories proposed that Africans didn't get sick because of their "thick skins" and "offensive odors."

The real reason the Africans resisted malaria had to do with genetics, a concept as foreign to the Europeans of the time as airplanes or antibiotics.

Evolution tends to work on a slow schedule with *Homo sapiens*. An adaptation to fight malaria could only evolve in human populations that had been exposed to the disease for a long period of time. The West African peoples so often taken as slaves had descended from ancestors that had dealt with malaria since prehistory. Over many generations, a biological defense against malaria called sickle cell evolved in some of those ancestors.

Long before English colonists started their own slave trade farther north, malaria found its way out of the Caribbean and Central America to attack native tribes and to lie in wait for new waves of Europeans.

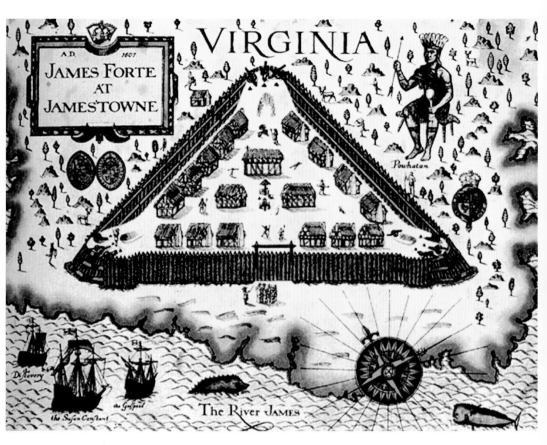

A map showing the fort at Jamestown, the early English settlement where 80 percent of immigrants died within a year of arriving due to starvation, wars with local tribes, and diseases like malaria.

Visit the former English settlement at Jamestown today and it's clean and quaint. In the early 1600s, Jamestown was one of the worst death traps in the New World. "Our men were destroyed with cruell diseases as Swellings, Flixes, Burning Fevers, and be warres," one colonist wrote.

From Jamestown's founding in 1606 through 1624, five out of every six colonists died of disease, depression, exhaustion, starvation, or wars with local tribes. Constant stress and over-work suppressed the colonists' immune systems, increasing their chances of catching illness. Even in the 1660s, 80 percent of new immigrants died within a year of their arrival. One Englishman declared Virginia and its marshy tidewaters, "thrice worse than Essex, Thanet, and Kent for agues and diseases . . . and standing water in the woods that bred a double corrupt air."

By the late 1600s, however, plantation owners in America were prosperous enough to need more workers. Unable to convince Europeans to perform agricultural labor, they adopted the Caribbean tradition of African slaves.

The Africans' sickle cell defense against malaria allowed the slaves to open up coastal areas of Virginia and the even more notorious Carolinas. Said one English proverb, "They who want to die quickly go to Carolina." Slave labor drained swamps for crops, particularly rice. But that wasn't the end of malaria. Rice farming requires paddies. *Anopheles* mosquitoes found that setting amenable to breeding. Malaria killed whites with such force that Carolinians seriously considered deserting Charles Town (today's Charleston) for safer ground.

Imported diseases like malaria often ran ahead of the Europeans themselves, spread by native tribes to one another via trade, wars, or other contact. Settlers and displaced Native Americans moving west also took swamp fever with them. River valleys in the interior swarmed with *Anopheles* mosquitoes. *Vivax* became a common colonial ailment; *falciparum* menaced a belt stretching from the warmer parts of the southeast to east Texas and into the valleys of the Ohio and Mississippi Rivers.

As far as we know, Europeans—and people unwillingly brought by Europeans—introduced malaria to the New World.

Early Spanish colonial writings do not mention *El paludismo*, and the Spaniards would have recognized a disease so common in their homeland. Had malaria existed in the Western Hemisphere before Columbus, it's probable that Native Americans would have developed genetic adaptations, the way Africans had with the sickle cell. But they had none. In fact, malaria, like all the diseases the Europeans imported, had a lethal effect on them. Coastal Mexican peoples already decimated by European smallpox and influenza may have been finished off by a malaria epidemic in the mid-1500s. As long as three centuries later, a California outbreak killed an estimated 30,000 Indians on the eve of the Gold Rush.

Yet among the New World's many mysteries was a remedy for malaria. In South America, Jesuit priests followed the conquistadors to the Andes. As they ministered, the missionaries discovered that native peoples treated fever with a tea brewed from the bark of a local tree. The bark would make fortunes and change history.

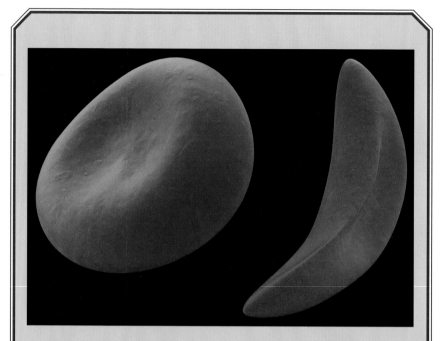

A rendering of a normal blood cell (left) and a sickle cell. *(Courtesy of Sebastian Kaulitzki/Alamy)*

SICKLE CELL ANEMIA

The sickle cell is named for the shape of the carrier's sickle-shaped red blood cells. Sickle cells prevent *Plasmodium falciparum* from reproducing enough to reach fatal levels in the bloodstream. Carriers can still catch *falciparum*. They just seldom die of it. The sickle cell cuts the chance of death by 90 percent.

Like many genetic adaptations, however, the sickle cell is itself a health hazard. A person inheriting the sickle cell gene from one parent is prone to anemia and to that condition's related health problems. Children who inherit the sickle cell gene from both parents tend to die young. Somewhere between 10 and 20 percent of Africans are carriers. Sickle cell-related problems also cause illness among African Americans and others of African ancestry.

three

The Fever Tree and the Magic Bullet

South America in the 1630s attracted many kinds of people: fortune hunters, entrepreneurs, ne'er-do-wells with few other options, and the odd explorer fascinated by the New World's alien flora and fauna. None approached life in the New World with more zeal than Jesuit priests. The Jesuits were members of the Society of Jesus, one of the church's youngest orders. They were dedicated to knowledge and missionary work, and filled with the dynamic energy common to idealists of all beliefs, spiritual and otherwise.

As Spanish colonies became established in Peru, Ecuador, and elsewhere, the Jesuits became an influential part of colonial life. They took special interest in ministering to the Native American survivors of the Spanish conquest. As they went about their missionary work, the priests learned native ways—the languages, food and drink, and medicine. Andean peoples, they found out, used a type of tree bark to calm the shaking associated with chills. Some locals called it *ayac cara,* or "bitter bark," because of its sharply bitter taste. It was better known as *quinaquina,* the "bark of barks," but it became famous as *Cinchona.*

The Jesuits welcomed the possibility of relief. Exotic New World parasites brought on fevers and chills aplenty in the New World, not all caused by malaria. Furthermore, many Jesuits had in the course of their careers passed through malarial Rome on visits to the Vatican. In the 1600s, as in ancient times, the Roman disease remained a leading cause of misery in the Holy City. No less than four popes had died of it in the century after 1492.

The Jesuits traveled widely, and soon word spread of a new fever remedy nicknamed Jesuit's bark. Some accounts credit Agostino Solumbrino, a Jesuit living in Lima, Peru, with sending the first samples of it to the Vatican in the early 1630s. Not long after, a local cardinal started dispensing free bark from a church hospital. The Jesuits, meanwhile, moved on the profit potential. The Society of Jesus took control of the bark trade, purchasing the product from natives in South America and reselling it to markets in Spain and Italy. Demand for the bark from the "fever tree" boomed.

The *Cinchona* tree is closely related to the coffee plant. In general it grows in hot climes on the eastern slopes of the Andes from Venezuela to Bolivia. It does particularly well in the rich soil on the sides of volcanoes at altitudes ranging from 4,000 to 10,000 feet above sea level. Some species grow as a bush, others as a tree. The tallest can reach fifty feet high. Like coffee, the *Cinchona* flowers

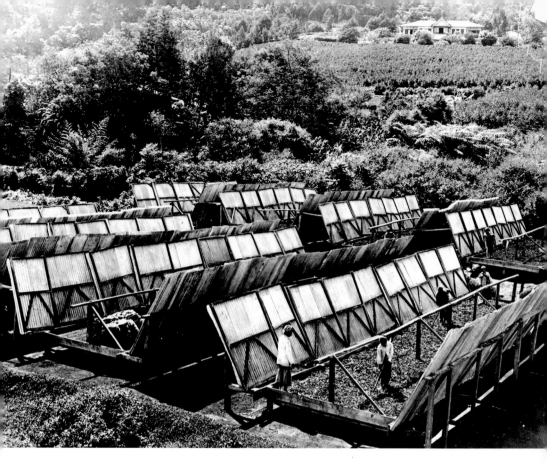

Quinine is the active antimalarial ingredient in *Cinchona* bark. In this 1960 photo, *Cinchona* bark dries in the sun so it can be pulverized for quinine production. *(Courtesy of Three Lions/Getty Images)*

and drops its fruit in short seasons that vary greatly, with weather conditions an important factor.

It soon became clear there were dozens of species of the tree, and that the medicinal effects of each kind of bark varied. To further confuse matters, *Cinchona* crossbred easily with other kinds of *Cinchona*, creating innumerable hard-to-identify hybrids. Some were a potent anti-malarial treatment. Others were useless.

Though unknown at the time, indeed unknown until chemistry became an established science, the bark's effectiveness depended on its quinine content. Quinine is the active anti-malarial ingredient, an alkaloid that when separated from the bark appears as white crystals. Quinine prevents the four malaria parasites from breaking into red blood cells. It's also a natural fever-reducer—it brings down body temperature by as much as three degrees—and muscle-relaxant. The Andean tribes had used it to treat fever and chills of various kinds long before they came into contact with malaria.

Quinine comes with a considerable downside, however. Side effects include intense headaches, nausea, and ringing in the ears.

Cinchona bark faced intense competition in the marketplace. Europeans often preferred their traditional cures—like wrapping a spider in rags and wearing it around the neck. Turquoise was also considered effective. Physicians, meanwhile, cast suspicion on the new medicine because it conflicted with accepted theories—most of which hadn't changed in a thousand years. Rural people preferred their own wide range of solutions. One cure for malaria was to bring a sheep to the patient's bedside to encourage the sickness to leave the person and jump into the animal.

Religious prejudice was an even more powerful deterrent. This was the era of Europe's bitter religious wars between Catholics and Protestants. Between 1618 and 1648, a devastating conflict that became known as the Thirty Years War engulfed central Europe. At the time that Solumbrino sent bark to Rome, the Thirty Years War, and the famines and epidemics related to it, was turning Europe into a wasteland.

Hatred blinded reason and eclipsed common sense. Protestants instinctively mistrusted any product connected to Catholics in general, and the zealous Jesuits in particular.

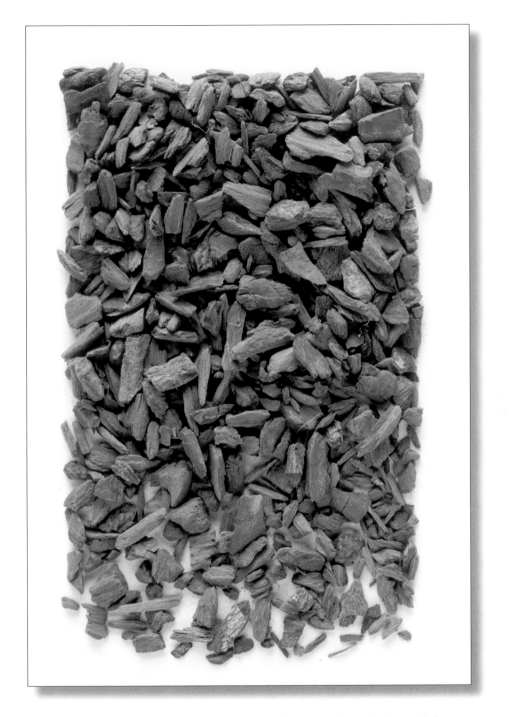

Dried bark from a *Cinchona* tree. In the 1600s, Jesuit missionaries learned that the native South American population used the bark from the *Cinchona* tree to relieve the fever and chills associated with malaria. *(Courtesy of Getty Images)*

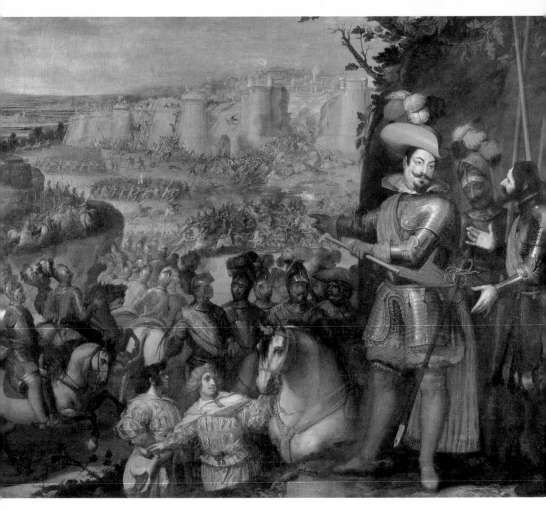

A 1634 painting of a battle during the Thirty Years War, a religious war between Catholics and Protestants. During this time, Protestants in Europe fostered an inherent distrust of any product associated with Catholics, including quinine.

According to legend, Oliver Cromwell, the Puritan leader of England, refused Jesuit bark while ill with the malaria that contributed to his death. When he died in 1658, England was suffering from the second major malaria epidemic in twenty years. Yet suspicion of all things Catholic was so strong that quinine was banned in the country and circulated only via the Catholic black market.

Then as now, one man's crisis is another's opportunity. English entrepreneur Robert Talbor saw his and seized it. Though considered a quack by the medical establishment, Talbor made a fortune selling a secret mixture for the *ague*. In a stroke of marketing savvy, Talbor hinted at quinine's worthlessness while at the same time refusing to give out the ingredients he used—one of which was quinine. He mixed the drug with wine to disguise its bitter taste.

Talbor's reputation grew, until in 1678, he treated no less than King Charles II for fever. To the horror of respectable physicians, Talbor cured the monarch. Charles made him a royal physician and knighted him. Soon Talbor was across the English Channel treating French royals sick with Paris's annual summer fever. One of them was King Louis XIV's son. Impressed by his heir's recovery, the king bought the secret recipe from Talbor for 3,000 gold crowns and a lifetime pension. Upon Talbor's death he had it published.

Cinchona bark thereafter became a part of Europe's collective medicine chest. But strangely enough, few Europeans—if any—had seen the fever tree with their own eyes.

Jose Celestino Mutis, a pioneering natural historian, studied the *Cinchona* for decades and advocated further scholarship in the name of knowledge and profit. "America is rich," he wrote the Spanish king, "there is quinine, a priceless possession of which Your Majesty is the only owner and which divine Providence has bestowed upon you for the good of mankind. It is indispensable to study the *Cinchona* tree so that only the best kind will be sold to the public at the lowest price."

But any man looking to make a fortune in *Cinchona* bark faced a daunting journey. First he had to avoid shipwreck,

The title page to Robert Talbor's secret malaria treatment, which he sold to King Louis XIV on the condition that it not be published until after his death.

yellow fever, scurvy, and starvation on the way to South America.

Then, if he chose to explore from the north via Colombia, he had to navigate rivers in malarial jungles inhabited by *Anopheles darlingi*—a mosquito so tough it could supposedly bite through leather.

Taking the west-to-east approach, however, presented him with the jagged Andes, the world's second-highest mountain range. While crossing the mountains he faced blizzards and glaciers, even rumbling volcanoes. Once on the eastern side, the explorer picked his way into cloud forests below—the home of deadly parasites, hostile tribes, and dangerous wildlife of all descriptions. Assuming his guides were competent and loyal, and if he didn't starve, he still faced the local bark hunters—the *cascarilleros*—who guarded the *Cinchona* to protect their own profits.

Regardless of an individual's bravery or determination, the *Cinchona* remained hard to find, let alone strip of its bark. The Europeans who succeeded had notably bad luck transporting seeds and seedlings out of South America. An uncanny number of samples burned up in fires or sank in shipwrecks. Often the seeds refused to grow in soil outside its habitat, or the trees turned out to be unprofitable, quinine-poor species.

As time passed, native chincona with quality bark became harder and harder to find. Not surprisingly, considering the money at stake, *cascarilleros* stripped too many trees. The Jesuits had tried to get them to plant five *Cinchona* trees (in the shape of a cross) for every one cut down. But the lesson never caught on.

By the early 1800s, it seemed possible the *Cinchona* might be hunted to extinction. The German explorer and naturalist Alexander von Humboldt guessed that 25,000 trees per year were killed just in Ecuador. The process accelerated in South America throughout the 1800s as Europe bought more and more bark.

Worried, European governments slowly came around to the idea of growing their own in tropical colonies. By doing so they hoped to guarantee a reliable supply at steady prices. The question was, which *Cinchona* should be grown?

Chemistry provided some clues.

In 1820, French chemists separated quinine from yellow-bark *Cinchona*. Manufacturers were soon processing the bark on a mass scale. As quinine became more widely available the price came down. But the bark available for manufacturing was so-so in quality. Chemists and capitalists raced to identify which species of *Cinchona* carried the most quinine. It was known that so-called red barks worked reasonably well. But the rare yellow barks had the richest quinine content and therefore the greatest value.

A new wave of nineteenth-century explorers set out in search of *calisaya*, a valuable yellow bark variety fiercely guarded by both *cascarillos* and South American governments. Its quinine-rich bark would change history. The two men responsible for bringing it to the world were Charles Ledger, an English fortune hunter, and Manuel Incra Mamani, a Bolivian *casarillero* and Ledger's business partner.

Ledger came to South America at age eighteen,

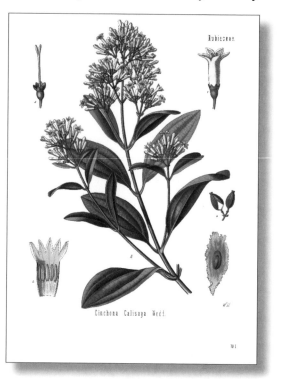

An illustration of the different parts of the *Cinchona calisaya*, a variety of *Cinchona* valued for its quinine-rich bark.

determined to get rich. First working for a trading house, then in business for himself, he learned all he could about *Cinchona*. Hearing of untapped trees in remote parts of Bolivia, Ledger courted native contacts in the region. It took caution. In Peru, a state-sponsored monopoly controlled the legal trade, leaving Ledger with no choice but to use smugglers. Bolivia guarded it even more fiercely. In the mid-1800s *Cinchona* bark was its top crop, and one the poor nation could not afford to lose.

A group of Peruvian businessmen interested in getting around the local monopoly hired Ledger to find the *calisaya*. Ledger brought Mamani as a guide and led a caravan of fifty-five smugglers into the interior. Mamani's knowledge of the *Cinchona* was profound. In time he started to share his expertise with his partner, and finally let it be known that the best *calisaya* grew on specific mountainsides in the Andes. (Mamani also explained how the locals sterilized *Cinchona* seeds so that Europeans could not establish their own plantations elsewhere.)

While on a scouting mission the two men stumbled onto a grove of fifty high-quality *Cinchonas*. It was the wrong time of year to take bark or seeds. But Ledger did not forget the grove of yellow-barked *calisaya*.

Ledger eventually went bankrupt on another moneymaking scheme, this one involving alpacas. Still determined to get rich, he used his last funds to send Mamani back into Bolivia in search of top-grade *calisayas*. For four straight years frost destroyed the *Cinchona* seeds before Mamani could harvest them. Finally, in 1865, he returned to Ledger with forty pounds of seeds. Ledger sent half to his brother in London, confident he was about to become a rich man.

But the British expressed little interest. They already grew *Cinchona* in India, their profitable Asian colony. Though the Indian trees were of inferior quality, the British appeared satisfied with what they had. Desperate, Ledger's brother contacted the Dutch government. The Dutch purchased a pound with an option to buy more if the seeds proved able to grow on their struggling quinine plantations in Java, part of their colony in the Dutch East Indies.

The Dutch's modest purchase changed everything. Research showed the *calisaya* to be a previously unknown species. The trees from Mamani's seeds yielded far more quinine than the low-quality species the Dutch had been growing. The mature bark contained 14 percent quinine, far more than any competitor. Once the *Cinchona* started producing, the Java plantations gave the Dutch a huge boost within the quinine industry. In time they dominated it. Botanists honored Ledger by naming the quinine-rich tree *Cinchona ledgeriana*.

Greater supplies brought down prices. Millions of malaria victims could now afford treatment. The result was a boost to public health around the world. Humanitarians applauded. European governments, by and large, appreciated quinine for other, less idealistic, motives. In the second half of the century, the European powers were racing to secure colonies rich in raw materials. Those regions were, almost inevitably, tropical and malarial.

Europeans for a long time had looked at Africa eagerly. Eagerly, that is, until they caught one of the continent's diseases. This reversed what the Europeans were used to. Relatively few new diseases had greeted European colonists in the New World. None stopped their advance. At the same

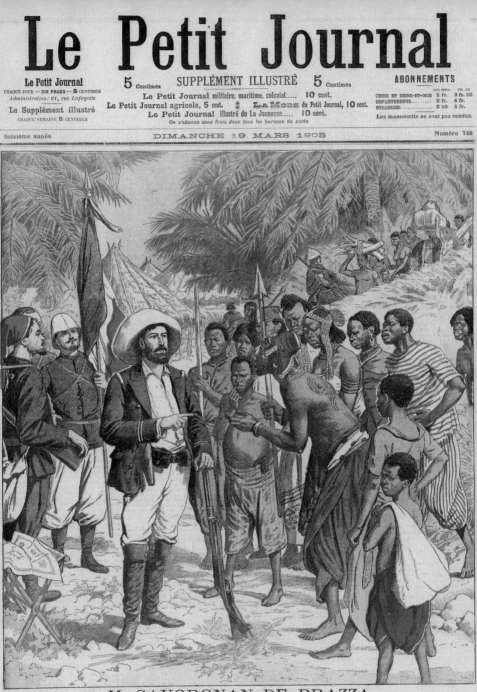

Le Petit Journal

Le Petit Journal
CHAQUE JOUR — SIX PAGES — 5 CENTIMES
Administration: 61, rue Lafayette

Le Supplément illustré
CHAQUE SEMAINE 5 CENTIMES

5 Centimes **SUPPLÉMENT ILLUSTRÉ** 5 Centimes

Le Petit Journal militaire, maritime, colonial..... 10 cent.
Le Petit Journal agricole, 5 cent. ❋ **LA MODE** du Petit Journal, 10 cent.
Le Petit Journal illustré de La Jeunesse..... 10 cent.
On s'abonne sans frais dans tous les bureaux de poste

ABONNEMENTS

	SIX MOIS	UN AN
SEINE ET SEINE-ET-OISE	2 fr.	3 fr. 50
DÉPARTEMENTS	2 fr.	4 fr.
ÉTRANGER	2 50	5 fr.

Les manuscrits ne sont pas rendus.

Seizième année **DIMANCHE 19 MARS 1905** Numéro 748

M. SAVORGNAN DE BRAZZA
Le vaillant explorateur au milieu de son escorte pendant son dernier voyage au Congo

A 1913 illustration of European adventurers and their guides exploring the Congo river region in Africa. Due to the constant presence of malaria in Africa, quinine was essential for European exploration of the continent. *(Courtesy of Mary Evans Picture Library/Alamy)* time, their own diseases did more than anything else to wipe out the original Native American inhabitants.

Malaria, however, provided Africans with a powerful line of defense. The sickle cell and constant exposure to the endemic malaria gave them a measure of immunity to local strains of the disease, whereas any European venturing more than a mile or two from the coastline invited death.

Scotsman Mungo Park took forty-four men down the Niger River in 1805. He brought back four, himself included. Malaria, crocodiles, and Africans killed the rest. Over the next few decades the British nonetheless established tenuous outposts, always within sight of the ocean. Soldiers posted to the Bight of Benin suffered tremendous death rates from disease. Official statistics showed the average soldier in 1840 went to the hospital for malaria three times a year. Not for nothing was Africa nicknamed the white man's grave.

The European exploration of Africa would have been impossible without quinine. The Baikie Expedition, above all others, encouraged the British to take it seriously as a preventative medicine.

An exploratory journey set out to explore the Niger, viewed as the most important of central Africa's river routes. While on the way the expedition's leader died. Rather than turn for home, William Balfour Baikie, the highest-ranking government officer on the ship, took command, despite the fact he had never been to Africa. Baikie had an obsessive belief in quinine. On his orders the not-always-appreciative crew took a dose of the drug twice a day. Baikie agreed to let it be dissolved in sherry to make it more pleasant. The expedition made it farther up the Niger than any previous attempt. No member of his crew, European or African, died of malaria.

Drug quality and the amount to take, however, remained serious issues. Many African explorers self-medicated, with varying success. Henry Stanley only survived numerous bouts with fever thanks to a drink he called the Zambesi Rouser—a quinine-spiked brew he took with water. Fellow explorer Richard Burton used an inadequate quinine-opium-sloes medicine and kept getting sick.

As with slavery centuries before, attitudes toward Africans dovetailed with Europeans' need to morally justify their conquest of darker races. Colonization became more than mere economic exploitation of African raw materials. Europeans also claimed they were bringing civilization to dark-skinned and savage barbarians.

The colonizers clearly saw disease as the Africans' ally. As the mania for colonies rose, advocates spoke of disease as a deadly enemy blocking economic, spiritual, and scientific progress. Their own, in particular. Some years later the famed malariologist Ronald Ross wrote, with the condescending racism typical of the time:

> Malarial fever . . . haunts more especially the fertile, well-watered and luxuriant tracts. There it strikes down not only the indigenous barbaric population but, with still greater certainty, the pioneers of civilization—the planter, the trader, the missionary and the soldier. It is therefore the principal and gigantic ally of Barbarism. . . . It has withheld an entire continent from humanity—the immense and fertile tracts of Africa.

As in the New World, this so-called progress worked very much in favor of Europeans. Africans lost their fertile tracts of native crops in favor of cash crops like coffee and cocoa. They were virtually enslaved to dig diamonds for British cor-

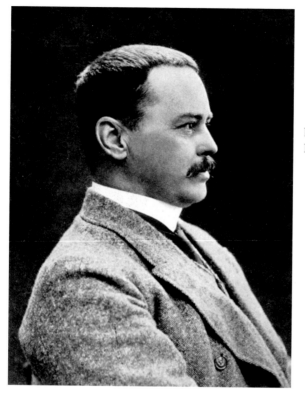

British physician
Ronald Ross.

porations or harvest rubber for the Belgian king. They died
by the millions of mistreatment and new diseases, and they
saw their lives and cultures uprooted and destroyed.

Europeans for the most part still congregated on the
coasts, as in French Algeria or British West Africa. Locals
and colonists rarely lived side by side. In Africa and India,
whites built mini-versions of European towns on high ground,
and strictly controlled disease within these enclaves according to the latest information from the experts.

Those experts usually worked in institutions specifi-
cally founded to facilitate colonial efforts in the tropics. The
British, having the largest colonial holdings, took a special

interest in the problem. Schools devoted to tropical medicine opened in London and Liverpool. As the European powers raced to claim chunks of Africa, it became imperative to understand the exotic diseases they encountered. Profits and national pride depended on it.

The idea of a relationship between mosquitoes and malaria was controversial, but it wasn't new. In 1854, the French-West Indian physician Louis Daniel Beauperthuy, having studied malaria in Venezuela, said:

> Intermittent fever is a serious disease spread by and due to the prevalence of mosquitoes. . . .[It owes its] toxicity to an animal or vegetoanimal virus, the introduction of which into the human system occurs by inoculation. The poisonous agent, after an incubation period, sets up . . . decomposition of the blood.

Years later, Albert King—the doctor famous for treating Lincoln at Ford's Theater—gave nineteen reasons proving the link. City fathers in Washington, D.C., still turned down his plan to build a giant wire screen around the capital.

As the century progressed and colonies became an integral part of European economies, a pair of physicians serving in areas overseas filled in many of the blanks. One was French, one British.

Louis Alphonse Laveran was a third-generation army doctor. Posted to an Algerian French Foreign Legion outpost in 1878, Laveran took an interest in malaria, an ailment he treated constantly. While treating a Legionnaire for an unusually persistent case of the disease, he made an unexpected discovery.

Laveran put a blood sample from his patient on a glass microscope slide. For some reason he waited or was

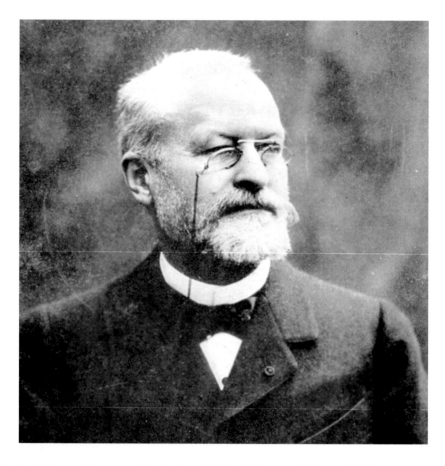

Louis Alphonse Laveran, the doctor who first discovered that malaria was caused by a parasite.

delayed for fifteen minutes—just enough time to allow the *falciparum* parasite on his slide to begin reproduction. When he returned to the microscope he became the first person to see the elusive malaria parasite.

"I was astonished," he wrote, "to observe at the periphery of this body was a series of fine transparent filaments that moved very actively and beyond question were alive."

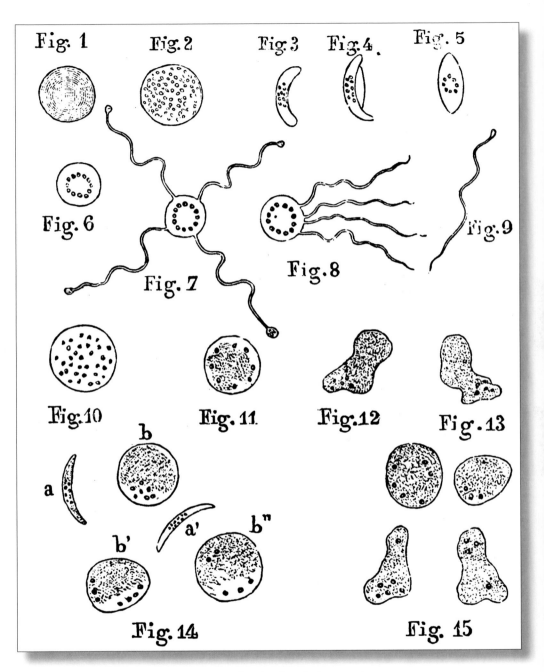

Laveran's 1880 sketch of malaria parasites.

Laveran's news that a parasite caused malaria failed to shake the world. The medical establishment ignored his finding. Leading malaria researchers insulted him and his subsequent research. It took four years and better microscopes before anyone took him seriously.

The parasite's complicated life cycle and changing shapes led subsequent research down a series of false trails. After the basic science was ironed out, a vital question remained: how did the parasite get inside human beings?

Ronald Ross did not appear qualified to solve the problem. While in medical school in London he preferred poetry or teaching himself mathematics to studying. He graduated at the lowest level possible one could graduate at and still call oneself a doctor. After that he spent several bored years as a physician in India.

On the brink of giving up medicine, he met Patrick Manson, a famed expert in tropical diseases then living in London. Inspired by their talks, the eccentric, though energetic, Ross returned to India and threw himself into malaria research.

Incredibly, he dreamed of making medical history while understanding next to nothing about his chosen work. Most of the leading malaria research was in languages he couldn't read. He barely knew how to use a microscope. Not only was he unaware of new techniques in staining microscope slides—a revolutionary tool in medical research—he had the barest knowledge of the *old* techniques. Most astonishing of all, Ross was completely ignorant about mosquitoes, including how to tell one species from another.

After studying the wrong kinds of mosquitoes for months, Ross by chance received ten *Anopheles* caught by an assistant. As he had done so many times, he fed the unfamiliar

Anopheles on a malaria patient. Over the next four days he dissected or ruined eight of the ten, and found nothing. On day four, however, he saw a telltale cyst in one mosquito's stomach—evidence that the parasite bred in the gut of the insect.

Other scientists began investigating the various aspects of the parasite's life cycle. Ross and a team of Italians, working separately but along parallel lines, traced the journey of the thread-like sporozoites in an *Anopheles*' saliva glands. Insects so infected passed on malaria to birds. Other experiments showed the same result with human subjects. Humanity's understanding of the man-mosquito-parasite cycle was complete.

Ross became world famous and won the 1902 Nobel Prize in Medicine. He lived out his years consulting on malaria control, composing poetry about disease, and writing memoirs to settle scores with his scientific rivals.

With mosquitoes revealed as the malaria vector, control of the insects took high priority. One of the first large-scale tests of this new direction took place in Panama. There, the United States was involved in one of the largest landscape-altering projects of all time—building a canal to link the Pacific Ocean with the Atlantic.

Yellow fever and malaria had already foiled an earlier French attempt to build a canal across Panama. When the U.S. took over, both diseases still killed or sickened huge numbers of workers. Desperate for results, the government called in an army doctor named William Crawford Gorgas, the leader of a successful mosquito control campaign in Cuba.

Gorgas put a series of anti-mosquito measures in place. On his order, trained workers covered water-collection sources

The page in Ronald Ross's notebook where he recorded the discovery of a cyst in a mosquito's stomach that he later identified as malaria parasites.

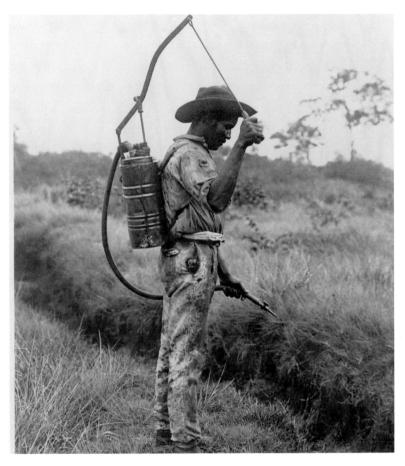

A worker killing mosquito larvae by spraying oil on open water near a Panama Canal work site. *(Library of Congress)*

with screens, drained ditches, and poured oil on open water to suffocate the mosquito larvae. Sprayers with pyrethrum, an insecticide made from chrysanthemum, fumigated the buildings used as housing for the workers. Yellow fever was declared eliminated in 1906.

Malaria proved more difficult. Gorgas countered by order-ing everyone to take a 150-milligram dose of quinine twice per day. Those workers objecting to the bitter taste could drink theirs in extra sweet pink lemonade. Gorgas overrode complaints about cost and efficiency and ordered screens be installed over windows in the workers' quarters. Workers were given bed nets to sleep under. Gorgas even paid West Indians to patrol barracks and catch or swat any mosquitoes.

After his controls were in place, Gorgas admitted malaria still caused more illness than all other local diseases put together. But cases were halved in three years and the rate continued to drop after that. In 1914, the year the canal opened, only fourteen people died of the disease.

The Panama program showed that getting the disease under control required attacking on several fronts—with quinine, anti-mosquito programs, nets and screens, and by removing sick patients so they would not be bitten again and spread the disease. The world took notice, the United States included.

Though today we think of malaria as a tropical illness, it remained a major health problem in the U.S. well into the 1900s. In fact, no disease had a greater effect on American social life or economic development.

Fevers had been a fact of life for settlers from colonial times into the 1800s. "Those were trying times," recalled one Nebraska woman. "My brother had been working in a dairy in North Platte [Nebraska] and got malaria in 1887. . . . He was delirious and I often wondered how he lived. It was three months before he could walk." Laura Ingalls Wilder wrote about her family's battle with the disease in *Little House on the Prairie.*

Pioneers and immigrants unlucky enough to get sick sometimes turned to Dr. Sappington's Fever Pills. Before the Civil War, the pills could be bought for a dollar a box (for twenty-four

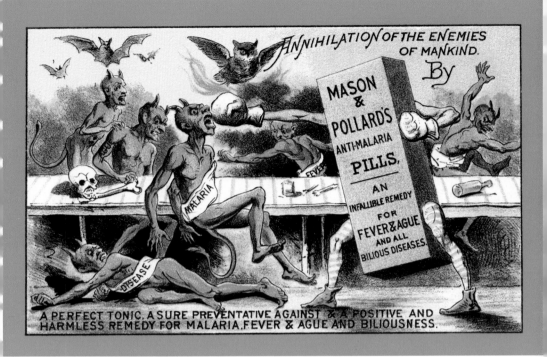

An early-1900s advertisement for anti-malaria pills. *(Courtesy of Paris Pierce/Alamy)*

pills). Sappington wisely mixed in licorice to cover up the quinine's taste. In its heyday the company turned out half a million boxes per year, until the Civil War drastically reduced quinine supplies in the U.S.

Soldiers on both sides could have used the pills. Malaria caused 10,000 deaths during the war. The Union blockade of the Confederacy ensured no quinine got in to help Southern soldiers, either.

In the first decades of the twentieth century, at least 5 million Americans per year suffered from new or recurring malaria. Twenty percent of the people in Staten Island, New York, carried it in 1900. Only a seven-year anti-mosquito program solved the problem and transformed Staten Island from malarial marsh into valuable real estate.

Without a doubt, however, malaria hit hardest at the southern states. In 1919, the U.S. Public Health Service said that "for the South as a whole it is safe to say that typhoid fever, dysentery, pellagra, and tuberculosis, all together, are not as important as malaria."

The South's hot and humid climate played a part, but poverty was the main issue. Southern cities, let alone rural areas, lacked the money for anything like the public works program on Staten Island. At the same time malaria hampered the economy. Industry refused to locate factories in the South because companies knew they'd lose workers for two to four weeks per year. And that was just to malaria. Even a malarial worker able to stay on his feet would be drained of energy or otherwise handicapped for long periods by the illness or the medicine. "I suffered with malaria for a period of two years and finally [overcame] it with quantities of quinine," said one Florida man. "It [the quinine] made me deaf as a post at the time, and turned my hair white."

During World War I, the Rockefeller Foundation, a charity organization dedicated to the eradication of disease, began partnering with Southern communities on malaria control. In ten years, Southern cities were almost clear at an estimated cost of forty-five cents per person. Other programs and local efforts pushed the disease out of the Great Plains, New England, and the upper Mississippi Valley. But it held on in the Tennessee River Valley and among the sharecroppers of the Mississippi Delta. That malaria clung to those strongholds was no surprise. Both places had undergone major ecological damage, usually for agriculture. Both places were also unusually poor.

Pharmaceutical companies, meanwhile, continued to look for a synthetic substitute for quinine. For all its usefulness, the traditional drug—now in its third century of use—fell short in ways beyond making people deaf. It quelled malaria's fever and the chills, but it didn't eliminate the parasites. And as long as the malaria *Plasmodium* was in the body, the disease could be transmitted. In Panama, for example, malaria had remained a threat because workers still carried parasites in their blood. Quinine also failed to get at *vivax* or *ovale* parasites hiding in the liver.

World War II created a military need for a new drug. Strategists foresaw that much of the war would be fought on tropical or subtropical battlefields in malaria hot spots like Sicily, the Philippines, and the South Pacific. Unfortunately for the Allies, Japan had invaded Java early on. Doing so gave the Japanese control of the Dutch chinchona plantations and 90 percent of the world's quinine supply.

Needing a solution, the military turned to Atabrine, a synthetic drug developed in 1930 but shelved because of toxic side effects. Atabrine had one important advantage over quinine. It interrupted the cycle that spread malaria by destroying the reproductive-stage parasites in the blood. That prevented the parasite from migrating to mosquitoes.

Soldiers had their doubts about Atabrine, especially when they found out it turned their skin bright yellow. Vomiting and diarrhea further subtracted from its reputation. There was also a false rumor that it caused impotence, and a truer one that on rare occasions it brought on temporary insanity.

Early in the war, superiors preoccupied with battlefield matters overlooked the need to make their troops take the medicine. The mistake struck home when U.S. forces invaded

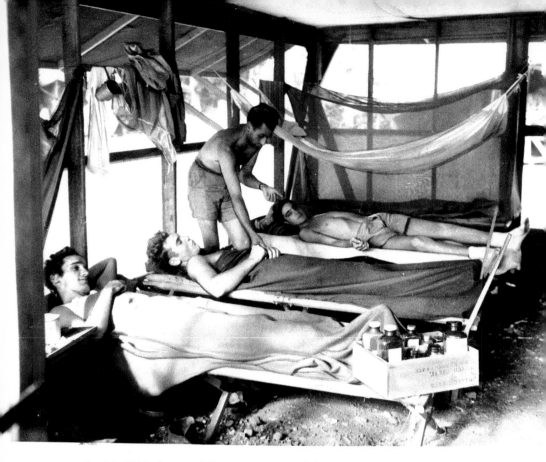

In this 1943 photo, soldiers recover in a field hospital after contracting malaria in Guadalcanal during World War II. *(Courtesy of AP Images)*

Guadalcanal, in the heavily malarial Solomon Islands. Eighty percent of the Marines came down with malaria, many of them with *falciparum*. Atabrine, fortunately, cured *falciparum*. But the drug had limits. It only held down the *vivax* parasite—it didn't get rid of it. Once a victim ceased treatment, the malaria surged back and again took him out of action.

General Douglas MacArthur wrote in 1943, "This will be a long war if for every division I have facing the enemy, I must count on a second division in hospital with malaria and a third division convalescing from this debilitating disease."

An order of April 18, 1943, laid out MacArthur's anti-malaria measures in detail. For the rest of the war U.S.

military personnel lined up and took their pills while watched by superiors. The British did the same. It wasn't always popular, but disciplined malaria control kept men in action and without a doubt contributed to the Japanese defeat.

It might have interested those GIs with yellow skin to know that a far superior, far less toxic drug sat in the archives of an American laboratory.

In 1934, the German corporation IG Farbin had developed and discarded a promising antimalarial called Resochin. At the time the German scientists dismissed it due to false worries about its side effects, but IG Farbin nonetheless shipped a Resochin sample to Winthrop Stearns, a sister company in the United States. Researchers at Winthrop Stearns promptly forgot about it.

The drug resurfaced during the war when the Allies liberated Tunis. French doctors showed Allied officers another IG Farbin antimalarial called Sontochin. American researchers chemically tweaked the new drug and named it chloroquine. As it turned out, chloroquine was identical to the discarded Resochin—the German researchers in the 1930s had made a mistake about the side effects.

Chloroquine acted by protecting red blood cells. Under normal circumstances, an iron-rich product in hemoglobin called heme is poison to the parasite. The parasite survives by turning heme into a nontoxic substance called hemozoin. Chloroquine prevented this process, leaving the helpless parasite to be poisoned.

The new drug was safe, far safer than Atabrine, and without any risk of insanity or diarrhea. In fact, the advantages seemed to solve a host of problems. Chloroquine acted fairly quickly, was easy to take and easy to manufacture, had a low

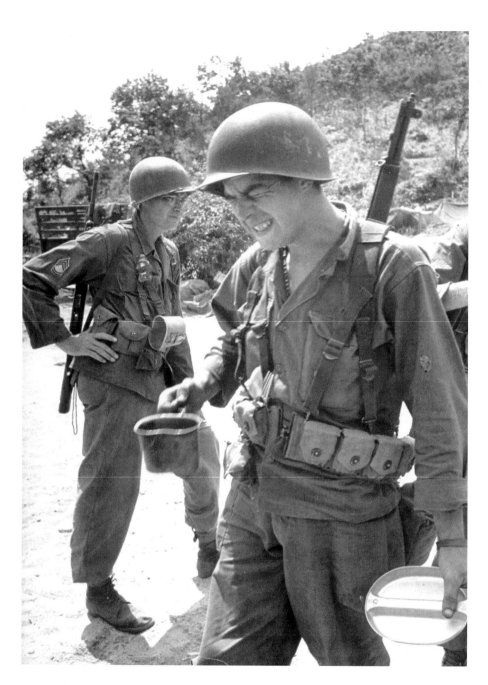

This Korean War soldier grimaces after taking a bitter chloroquine tablet. Chloroquine became one of the most famous drugs in the world after it was discovered that it could kill the malaria parasite in the human body. *(Courtesy of Joseph Scherschel/Time Life Pictures/Getty Images)*

price, and, being synthetic, eliminated the need to grow chinchona trees. In other words, it was too good to be true.

In a few years chloroquine would be one of the most famous drugs in the world, an astonishing lifesaver and a so-called magic bullet in the worldwide drive to eliminate malaria. Believers in the wonders of technology praised it as an ally to human progress alongside penicillin and the jet engine. In the years ahead, the magic bullet would be teamed with another miraculous discovery that had sat on a shelf for years. Chemists called the wondrous compound dichloro-dipheyl-trichloroethane. The world came to know it by the abbreviation DDT.

four
Eradication

Malaria fighters had employed chemicals ever since
William Gorgas used pyrethrum in Panama. The
first significant step up was Paris green, a copper-
arsenic poison deadly to mosquito larvae. Called "the most
important addition to our knowledge of malaria control in a
decade," Paris green was safe, cheap, and easy to apply—
sprayers only had to mix it with ordinary road dust before
spreading it on water where mosquitoes laid their eggs.

Paris green's effectiveness in Europe, particularly Italy,
encouraged the Rockefeller Foundation to change direction.
The disease-fighting institution turned away from malaria
treatment and research, and instead focused on mosquito control. "[T]he distribution of quinine . . . has never in any place
in any country been effective in controlling malaria," said
malaria-fighter Paul F. Russell. "[M]alaria control . . . must
consist mainly in a direct attack on the adult malaria-carrying

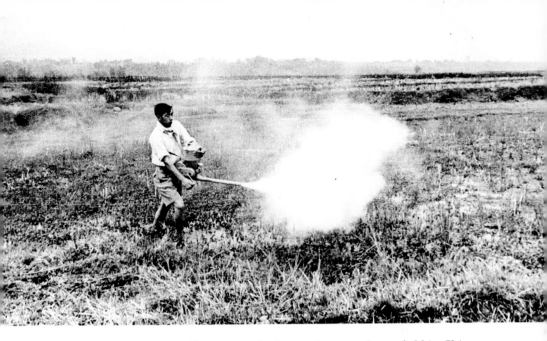

Paris green, a poison deadly to mosquito larvae, is sprayed on a field in China in this 1939 photo.

mosquito in its daytime resting places, or on the larva of this mosquito in its breed places, or on both at the same time."

But Paris green, for all its usefulness, only killed larvae. Public health experts needed an insecticide that killed adult, disease-transmitting mosquitoes.

In the late 1930s, chemist Paul Müller worked for the Swiss pharmaceutical company J. R. Geigy. While looking for a chemical to kill wool-destroying moths, Müller came across dichloro-diphenyl-trichloroethane (DDT), a chlorinated hydrocarbon discovered in 1874 by a chemistry student named Othmer Zeidler.

DDT worked on more than annoying moths. Tests on an infestation of Colorado potato beetles showed the chemical to be potent against a number of crop-destroying pests.

The Second World War engulfed Europe shortly after Müller's discovery. Subsequent interruptions in anti-malaria programs allowed the disease to surge back in parts of Europe.

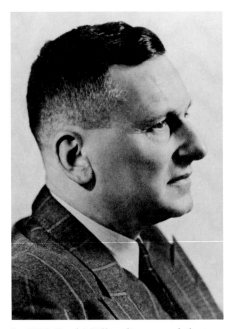

In 1939, Paul Müller discovered that DDT could be used to kill mosquitoes and a number of crop-destroying pests. *(Courtesy of Mary Evans Picture Library/Alamy)*

It hit especially hard in Italy. Over the previous twenty-five years the Italians had, with the help of the Rockefeller Foundation, committed to malaria control, from filling in ditches to use of Paris green to releasing fish that ate mosquito larvae. The government also drained the Pontine Marshes south of Rome. Notoriously malarial for centuries, the area became fertile farmland. By the war's outbreak, Italy had significantly reduced its malaria cases for the first time since the glory days of the Roman Empire.

The German Army reversed parts of the progress in an attempt to stop American and British troops. Taking a page from ancient history, the Germans flooded marshlands and turned loose millions of *Anopheles labranchiae*, a malaria vector. The crude attempt at biological warfare failed— American and British troops, unlike the Athenians, carried Atabrine. But the subsequent epidemic struck hard at Italian civilians.

Seeing the damage, and worried about a return to the bad old days, the Rockefeller Foundation decided to try out DDT on the country's thriving mosquito populations. Allied authorities in occupied Italy had already OK'd the chemical's use to destroy disease-carrying lice on war refugees. The positive results encouraged DDT production for the war effort. Secret factories began to turn it out by the ton.

The chemical brought dramatic results in Italy. *Anopheles* mosquitoes appeared defenseless; the number of malaria cases crashed wherever it was used. When the war ended, Foundation scientists proposed to use DDT to drive malaria from Italy and Sicily for good. In three years the disease that had frightened popes and troubled Italian farmers for more than ten centuries was almost gone. Only the rugged island

In this 1945 photo, DDT is being sprayed on an Italian house's interior walls in an effort to eradicate malaria. *(Courtesy of National Museum of Health and Medicine)*

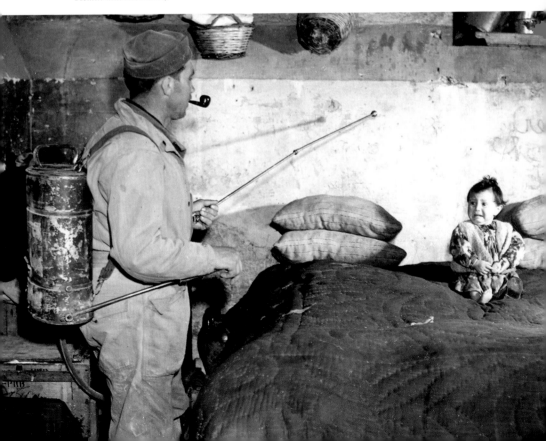

of Sardinia remained a reservoir. The Foundation's focused effort there employed Sardinians to drain swamps while it soaked the island with DDT. Malaria vanished.

Malaria fighters deployed DDT in a way that used a mosquito's habits against it. Everyone knew the female *Anopheles* settled on a nearby vertical surface after feeding. Since mosquitoes often fed indoors, DDT was sprayed on interior walls of houses. The female absorbed the chemical while it rested. The chemical's attack on its nervous system caused uncontrolled, fatal spasms long before the parasites inside the insect could mature.

To add to its effectiveness, DDT lasted up to six months, unheard of in an insecticide at the time. When Müller won the 1948 Nobel Prize in Physiology or Medicine, the presenting speaker told a story about the chemical in action:

> After the DDT solution had been sprayed on [the window], the flies died and lay in heaps on the window ledge. The following morning a German soldier entered and thoroughly cleaned the window. When the Major noticed this he couldn't help crying, "Goodbye, my DDT!" But this farewell was uncalled for. In spite of the thorough cleaning, the window pane retained its deadly action on the flies.

As the story suggests, people loved DDT because it wiped out aggravating insects like flies and lice. In fact, it killed *everything*—bedbugs, scorpions, spiders, lizards, even cockroaches. "The locals regarded this as the best thing that had ever happened to them," said Thomas Aitken, a Rockefeller Foundation worker in Sardinia. "The fact that malaria was gone was welcome. But also the DDT got rid of the houseflies. Sardinian houses were made of stone. The wires for the lights ran along the walls near the ceiling. And if you looked up at the wires they were black with housefly droppings from over the years. And suddenly, the flies disappeared."

No program got more dramatic results than the one in Ceylon (modern-day Sri Lanka), an island off southern India famous for its tea plantations. A deadly malaria epidemic in 1934-35 had killed more than 80,000 people. Authorities responded by starting a malaria surveillance service to watch for and curb mosquito breeding. Ceylon added DDT to its program in 1945. The death rate dropped by a quarter in one year. Over the next decade, Ceylon's conscientious anti-malaria program, using DDT as its main weapon, reduced cases from 3 million to just over 7,000, with zero malaria deaths reported.

From countries like the Netherlands and Taiwan to regions like the Caribbean orders poured in for the wonder chemical. The U.S. government allocated $7 million dollars to a spraying campaign. Magazine ads celebrated its killing power. Walt Disney made an educational cartoon that showed Doc and the rest of the Seven Dwarfs covering the insides of their huts with insecticide. A new government project, the Communicable Disease Center (later the Centers for Disease Control), was set up to deal with malaria once and for all. By the early 1950s, the government declared the disease gone from the U.S.

People hailed DDT, with some justification, as the atomic bomb of the insect world. Clearly, anything that could clear an age-old fever pit like Italy heralded a new era in fighting malaria, just as the A-bomb did when it came to wars of another kind.

DDT, however, played a secondary role in the U.S. and northern Europe. In those places, the environmental conditions that allowed mosquitoes to thrive had been changing for a long time. Malaria initially gained its hold centuries earlier because rampant deforestation turned the landscape into a good breeding ground. But by the 1900s the forests were long gone. Advanced agriculture had become well-established. Farmers took advantage of new technology—whether earth-moving machinery or Paris green—to deal with remaining malaria-producing marshes.

Such activities cost money. The countries that had it could escape malaria; the countries without suffered. It was no coincidence that wealthy Britain, able to pay to drain its eastern swamps and buy quinine, escaped the *ague* long before DDT came along. Mosquitoes thrived in southern Italy and Sardinia in part because those places were two of the poorest regions of a poor country. True, DDT appeared to have saved Ceylon. But some of the poorer Ceylonese lived in mud huts or tents—and they tended to carry the malaria that remained in the country.

The U.S. provided an excellent example of how wealth helped prevent malaria. New York and New Jersey, places with good economies and lots of taxpayers, could pay for anti-malaria measures in Staten Island and the Meadowlands. But while suburbanites built houses in those places, people in the Tennessee River Valley—too poor even to afford screens for their windows—continued to spend their summers languishing with fevers.

Historians and others interested in malaria differ over how much or how little DDT helped end America's malaria problem. Whatever the answer, the U.S. had already defeated malaria almost everywhere using medicine and mosquito control. To root it out of such strongholds as the Tennessee River

Valley took not only DDT, but investment in public works and education, and the prosperity that arose from both.

Starting in the 1930s, the Tennessee Valley Authority began to build hydroelectric dams in the region—a profound environmental alteration that nonetheless gave its engineers the power to control mosquito-breeding waters. Officials went house to house providing advice on how to avoid malaria.

Living standards slowly improved. The dams created cheap electricity, and the government provided the infrastructure

A 1942 photo showing the early stages of construction for Douglas Dam, a project of the Tennessee Valley Authority. Hydroelectric dams such as this provided cheap electricity for rural households, which in turn raised living standards and decreased the number of malaria cases in the area. (*Library of Congress*)

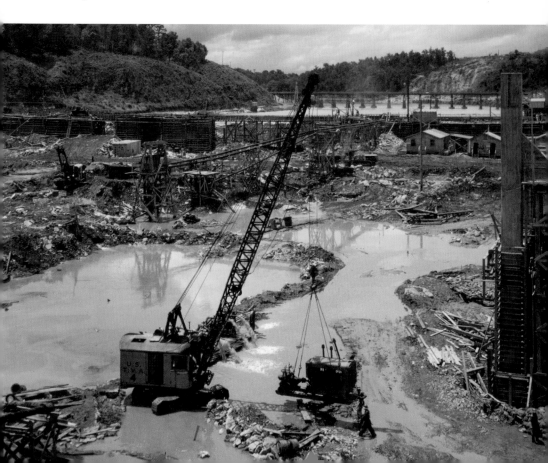

to carry it to rural people. World War II also brought better jobs to the area. Better jobs meant more disposable income for window screens and medicine. Economic improvement had already cut into malaria when the government started spraying DDT in the mid-1940s. The chemical certainly helped with mosquitoes. It also saved crops from other pests, giving farmers more to sell and thus more money. But in the end, DDT may have only sped up what was going to happen anyway.

A world of differences separated Ceylon from Sardinia, and rural Tennessee from the Pontine Marshes. But poverty and malaria, each contributing to the other, connected them all. One of DDT's subtle appeals was that it solved the malaria problem without having to address the far more complicated issue of how to improve the lives of the poor.

The U.S. government ceased spraying DDT for malaria around 1951. To everyone's surprise, the disease failed to return. The situation was the same in Crete, the Mediterranean island south of Greece. DDT plus generous handouts of chloroquine looked like the perfect strategy. An ancient killer was in full retreat.

But evolution's subtle machinery was also at work. The *Anopheles* mosquito began to resist DDT.

Greece turned to a DDT program after the war. Sprayers were trained to apply the chemical and, in an effort to enlist communities (and cut costs), were often fed and housed by the rural villages where they worked. Since DDT remained potent for up to six months, the spray men—in theory, at least—could get results treating every house once a year around mosquito-breeding season. Simultaneously, other spray teams, on foot or in airplanes, applied the chemical on ponds and other outdoor breeding areas.

In 1949, three years after the first sprayings, the local malaria vector *Anopheles sacharovi* began to change its behavior—a sure sign that something was up. Instead of biting and resting on the DDT-treated wall, *A. sacharovi* bit and then flew outside. Not long after, the chemical no longer harmed some mosquitoes. By 1951, the *A. sacharovi* and two other Greek species in certain areas sat on fresh DDT without any ill effects.

Experts understood what was going on. Intense use of DDT had weeded out mosquitoes vulnerable to it, leaving behind that part of the *Anopheles* population able to resist the chemical's effects. Biologists call the process selection pressure.

An initial DDT attack wiped out almost all of an area's *Anopheles* mosquitoes. But not quite all. The relatively few survivors lived because they carried a genetic mutation, an enzyme in their bodies that rendered the poison less toxic or even harmless.

At first the survivors weren't numerous enough to spread much malaria. Rates went down and victory seemed to be in sight. In time, though, these survivors bred with other survivors and passed along the mutation. The mutation-carrying offspring mated with other mutation-carrying mosquitoes, and so on. *Anopheles* can mate days after birth and create several generations of DDT-resistant insects quickly. While this was going on, the long-lasting DDT killed mosquitoes with imperfect mutations—leaving only the most resistant insects alive to breed.

Resistant mosquitoes, it turned out, could take over in as little as six years.

The World Health Organization (WHO), the public health arm of the United Nations, sent out a warning.

The scientific community, meanwhile, disagreed on what the Greek reports meant. Was it a local phenomenon only? A freakish occurrence? Or should tactics everywhere be changed? That mosquitoes in different places evolved resistance at different speeds confused the issue further.

In the meantime, DDT continued to be sprayed, not just for malaria, but in agriculture.

As it turned out, the reports from Greece were a warning. Resistance soon turned up elsewhere.

A 1956 WHO report stated, "There is . . . reason to fear that sooner or later repeated exposure of a community of Anopheles mosquitoes to DDT . . . will result in the development of strains which will either not be poisoned, or else will avoid contact with treated surfaces."

Fred Soper, an American malariologist, shared the view that if DDT was to destroy malaria, it had to happen before mosquito populations worldwide evolved resistance. Dictatorial and single-minded, and a natural-born leader, Soper was a legend in malaria circles. In 1938 he had taken charge of a Rockefeller Foundation effort in Brazil to wipe out *Anopheles gambiae*, an African species brought in on ships.

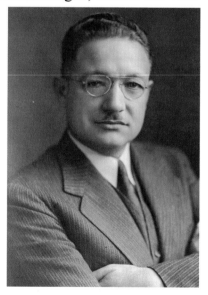

Fred Soper *(Courtesy of the National Library of Medicine, History of Medicine Division)*

A. gambiae is the world's most efficient malaria vector, able to breed in just about any muddy water, even rainwater inside a human footprint. It's also an aggressive biter of humans with a habit of carrying the *falciparum* parasite. When Soper presented his plan to kill every *gambiae* in Brazil, skeptics said wiping out such a resourceful insect was preposterous. Soper succeeded in just under two years.

As DDT resistance became a worry, Soper lobbied Marolino Candau, the WHO director-general, to launch the Global Malaria Eradication Programme—a one-time war to wipe malaria from the face of the earth.

Paul Russell, who had moved from the Rockefeller Foundation to Harvard, issued an influential report that put what was at stake in plain terms. "[I]f countries, due to lack of funds, have to proceed slowly, resistance is almost certain to appear and eradication will become economically impossible. *Time is of the essence* because DDT resistance has appeared in six or seven years. . . . This is a completely unique moment in the history of man's attack on one of his oldest and most powerful disease enemies."

The idea was that the WHO's organizational and medical expertise, along with the cooperation of local governments, would wage the kind of ruthless, highly disciplined eradication efforts pioneered by Soper in Brazil.

In an era in love with technology, and convinced it could conquer nature, the grand goal of eradicating malaria appeared possible. Humanity had harnessed the atom. Pilots had broken the sound barrier. The polio vaccine and recent discovery of DNA held out the promise of a healthier future. Surely even the mosquito, even this most ancient of diseases, couldn't stand against humanity's unified energy and intellect.

The Global Malaria Eradication Programme rolled out in 1957. The U.S. Congress promised to fund 31 percent of the WHO's total budget and 95 percent of the malaria effort, a massive amount of money equal to billions of dollars. In addition, poor countries to benefit from the program put up 35 percent of their health budgets. Congress promised to continue funding through 1963. The WHO's experts, using mathematical models, had determined that would be all the time necessary to finish the job.

The plan had three phases. The first was to drastically reduce malaria in a short time by killing mosquitoes with DDT. In places where the insects resisted DDT, programs would use other long-lasting pesticides. As in earlier campaigns, the WHO plan focused on structural interiors and outdoor breeding sites. Soper believed that spraying eight of ten houses would be enough to disrupt the malaria transmission cycle.

In phase two, authorities would provide chloroquine to clear malaria parasites from human beings. For places unable to get drugs, the program counted on *vivax* burning itself out in three years. The thinking was that even if DDT-resistant mosquitoes returned, no parasites would be left in human bloodstreams for them to drink up. The man-mosquito-parasite cycle would be broken. Malaria transmission would cease.

According to the experts' math, breaking the chain of transmission would take four years. *Anopheles* mosquitoes needed six years to evolve resistance to DDT. Since an area's malaria would be gone by the time that happened, the surviving mosquitoes would be nothing more than a buzzing annoyance on summer evenings.

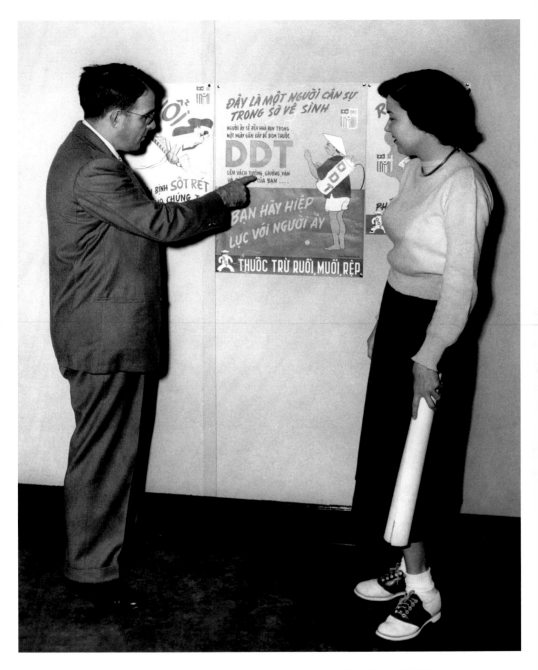

An employee for the Centers for Disease Control describes a DDT poster used in a malaria control program in Indochina. *(Courtesy of Centers for Disease Control and Prevention)*

During an ongoing final phase, each country would undertake surveillance measures to track conditions favorable to malaria's return. If cases appeared, trained teams could deal with it before the outbreak turned serious. The WHO would help where necessary.

From the Balkans to coastal North Africa, from western and southern Asia through tropical Australia and the South Pacific, sprayers set off to cover the walls of houses and huts with DDT.

A sprayer carried a pressurized tank on his back. Normally the container held three gallons of DDT powder mixed with water or, in some cases, oil. Not everyone was thrilled to see him at the door. They had to take down pictures from the walls and move furniture into the middle of the room. Food and eating utensils had to be carried outside.

The sprayer applied the DDT in an up-and-down pattern, covering the walls and ceiling before going outside to spray the eaves of the roof. Those living in the house had to wait a half hour for the chemical to dry. A faint chlorine smell hung in the air while they pushed the furniture back into place.

Reports of initial successes came in to WHO headquarters in Geneva. Sri Lanka once again encouraged high hopes. The country's case load fell from 3 million after WWII to a negligible number in 1962 and, finally, to a total of twenty-nine confirmed cases in 1964. The remaining victims tended to be poor citizens living in camps or people otherwise exposed to the elements.

To the north, India formed attack units, each responsible for a certain number of people. At one point almost four hundred of these teams patrolled the country, with 150,000 people employed overall in the field and in laboratories. Though the British had used DDT in the country as early as 1945, India carried an estimated 75 million cases in 1951. In ten years, the Indian government claimed the number was down to 50,000. While some observers considered the real number closer to 200,000, the larger figure still meant a 99 percent reduction.

The death of insect pests brought an increase in comfort, good health, and good crops to millions of people around the world—benefits that seemed worth the trouble of swallowing chloroquine or letting a sprayer in the door. Lands as diverse as Italy and Nepal opened up areas of farmland once too dangerous to use.

Optimism was so high that Harvard quit offering courses in malaria control. Malaria research everywhere all but stopped. Andrew Spielman, later a leading malaria expert, met with his guilt-stricken graduate school mentor and was told, "It's all over. There will be no career for you."

But by 1960 a growing number of experts had reservations about the campaign. Cracks in the program had appeared, in large part due to human failure.

Soper had shown in Brazil that an eradication campaign depended on conscientious, well-trained, well-led teams. The best inspectors and supervisors paid intense attention to detail and had a sure hand with the suspicious or annoyed townspeople.

In many countries, however, it was hard to find, let alone keep, the best employees. The repetitive nature of their jobs bored sprayers and lab technicians alike. Quality of training varied. So did commitment and leadership. In India, for example, the jobs were often filled by migrant workers with

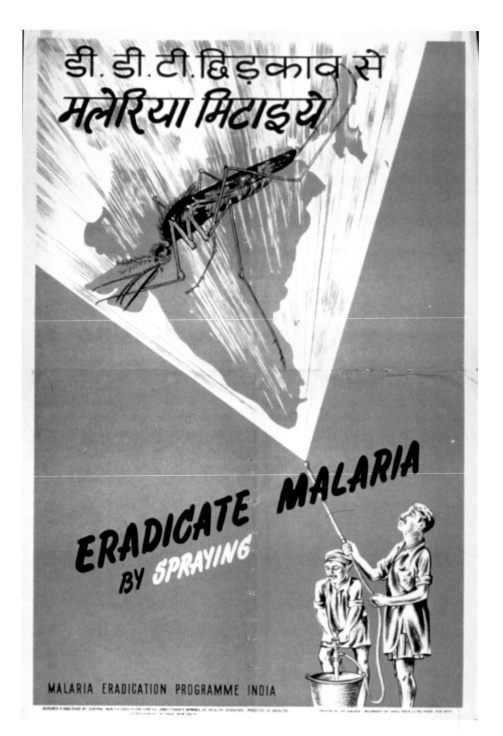

A 1960 poster from India depicts a man spraying a large mosquito with DDT. DDT was viewed as an integral part of the Global Malaria Eradication Programme's plan to eliminate malaria worldwide. *(Courtesy of the National Library of Medicine, History of Medicine Division)*

little connection to the region they sprayed or to the eradication program.

Inevitably, mistakes were made. Spraying took place at the wrong time of year, or in the wrong place, or in the wrong amounts, or not at all. The problem was that mosquitoes missed in one place caused disease elsewhere. Statistically, one infected person could spread enough parasites to spark an epidemic. Sicily's 1956 outbreak—thousands of cases— had started with *one* human carrier.

In a country like India, citizens were spread over gigantic areas. This posed challenges the campaign simply could not answer. Despite the huge effort, parasites remained in the blood of nomads, tribal groups, and remote communities. Mosquitoes could still pick up parasites from these people and, therefore, could still spread malaria.

To add to the problem, people in most of the stubbornly endemic countries started to get tired of spray men and medical tests. The program had dragged on longer than promised. They didn't want to hear about anti-malaria efforts anymore, or about the necessity for long-term surveillance.

As enthusiasm faded, questions became louder. Why spend precious money on a disease that was about to be eradicated? The surveillance phase cost as much as eradication—wasn't the WHO's program supposed to be a one-time expense? What about all the other problems—medical and otherwise—that needed attention?

Political leaders had to be sensitive to the public mood if they wanted to remain political leaders. As a result, many countries pushed malaria further and further down the government agenda. To make matters worse, the U.S. Congress, convinced eradication couldn't work, cut off funding after the WHO's 1963 deadline.

Nature presented an even more serious obstacle. In certain places chloroquine no longer affected *falciparum* parasites.

As early as 1960 there were reports of drug resistance in Colombia and Venezuela. Two years later the same thing occurred across Southeast Asia. In scientific terms the news made sense. The overuse of chloroquine had, inadvertently, applied the kind of selection pressure that was guaranteed to create a highly resistant parasite.

People throughout the malarial world had taken steady amounts of the drug for years. It was as common as aspirin in medicine cabinets. Poorer countries benefited from millions of tablets given away by the United States, particularly in India and Africa. A handful of well-intentioned nations added it to table salt to facilitate treatment.

Unfortunately, ongoing use of low doses failed to knock out the parasite. But the practice succeeded in encouraging it to evolve to resist the drug.

The United States experienced the developing drug resistance firsthand. In 1965, the U.S. was fighting a full-scale war in Vietnam. A nation of jungle, rice paddies, and river deltas, Vietnam was home to strains of drug-resistant malaria that hindered military operations and haunted soldiers. In some areas the infection rate soared to 60 percent. With chloroquine increasingly worthless, the U.S. military combined it with a new synthetic drug, primaquine, into the so-called CP tablet. Unfortunately, parasites developed resistance to CP in less than two years.

Chloroquine-resistant malaria soon spread throughout Asia. By the early 1990s, *falciparum* resisted the drug across

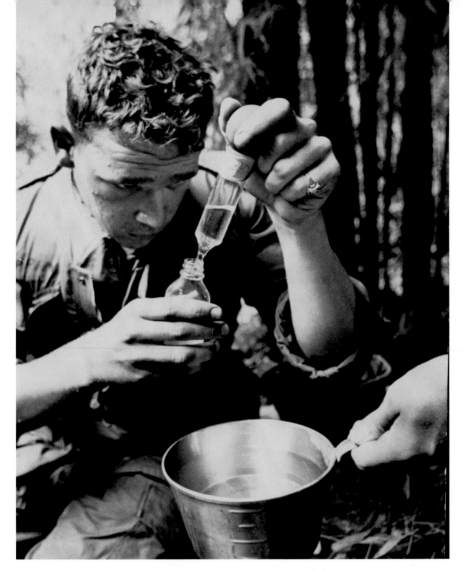

In this 1967 photo, a U.S. soldier in Vietnam puts *Anopheles* mosquito larvae in a test tube to be tested for malaria. *(Courtesy of Charles Bonnay/Time Life Pictures/Getty Images)*

the continent. In the meantime, resistant strains migrated to Africa. An unrelated resistant strain appeared in New Guinea.

Chloroquine's diminishing effectiveness warned of a future human tragedy. The overuse of DDT was an environmental disaster that already existed.

Today DDT is synonymous with environmental damage and pollution. Forty years ago it had a completely different image. Experts and ordinary people alike considered it a miracle on a par with the latest vaccines. The change in opinion came in large part because of a single book, Rachel Carson's *Silent Spring.*

Rachel Carson's book, *Silent Spring,* railed against the overuse of DDT and launched the environmental movement. *(Courtesy of U.S. Fish and Wildlife Service)*

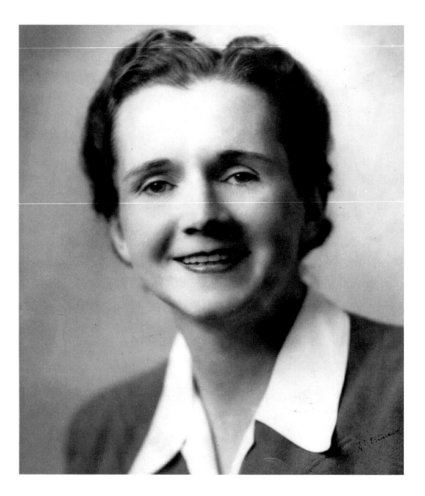

Carson began writing *Silent Spring* about the time the WHO launched the eradication campaign. In its pages Carson expressed concern that overuse of DDT had created a swarm of resistant disease vectors, not just for malaria, but for typhus and other serious illnesses carried by insects.

"The world has heard much of the triumphant war against disease through the control of insect vectors of infection," she said, "but it has heard little of the other side of the story—the defeats, the short-lived triumphs that now strongly support the alarming view that the insect enemy has been made actually stronger by our efforts. Even worse, we may have destroyed our very means of fighting."

Carson also saw a second, wider problem. DDT, she wrote, was responsible for catastrophic die-offs of fish, birds, and other wildlife. Being virtually nonbiodegradable, it lingered in animal tissue and collected in the liver, kidneys, adrenals, and sex organs. When DDT didn't poison the animal outright, the chemical often made it unable to reproduce. DDT and its harmful effects also continued up the food chain as predators ate toxic prey. In the most famous example, the eggs of bald eagles and other fish-eating species became so fragile they broke when sat on by the female birds.

More dramatically, Carson showed that DDT had found its way into wells, irrigation works, groundwater—and into human beings. Virtually every human being on earth, in fact.

Silent Spring was a bombshell. Despite scientists' and chemical companies' attacks on Carson, the book became a founding text of the environmental movement.

The relatively modest amount of DDT used for mosquito control wasn't the problem. Agriculture was another story.

Farmers used DDT's all-purpose killing power to wipe out any and all pests. Because the chemical was so cheap, American farmers bathed their fields in it. Poorer nations, where a bad harvest meant famine, couldn't resist using part of its donated DDT stock on crops instead of mosquitoes. In the mid-1940s, for example, a single season's spraying had boosted the Greek olive yield through the roof.

Carson didn't argue for a ban on DDT so much as against saturating fields and wilderness for pest control. As biologist C. J. Briegèr put it in her book, "Practical advice should be, 'Spray as little as you possibly can,' rather than, 'Spray to the limit of your capacity'. . . . Pressure on the pest population should always be as slight as possible."

But legal and political pressure to ban DDT snowballed throughout the 1960s. Malaria experts rightly pointed out that the environmental damage had nothing to do with their campaigns, that agriculture was to blame, and that DDT had saved millions of lives. Carson, they argued, had condemned DDT for the sins of all pesticides, many of which were far more toxic.

But she had laid out the case against DDT so dramatically that *Silent Spring* eclipsed the malariologists' arguments. In 1973, the Environmental Protection Agency banned DDT's use in the U.S. Other countries quickly followed.

By the time the ban took effect, the WHO had already declared defeat. The organization cancelled the eradication program in 1969 amidst bitter criticism of its methods. DDT's reputation as a miracle had faded for scientific reasons, as well. Almost forty *Anopheles* species resisted the chemical. Some mosquitoes could swim in it without harm.

Over the next decade, malaria became entrenched again across the tropics, with grim results.

The failure proved especially tragic in India. Having cut malaria by 99 percent a decade earlier, the country faced a million new cases in 1971. The government found it hard to find adequate money for programs because of the rising prices of pesticides other than DDT and the oil needed to mix them with. Furthermore, millions of Indians lacked any previous exposure to the disease because of earlier anti-malaria programs. When the mosquitoes returned, they fell ill in terrible numbers. By 1975, India was reporting 6 million cases.

Nor did Sri Lanka fare well. Having almost eradicated the disease, the country came under renewed assault. Anti-malaria efforts brought cases from over half a million down to 150,000. But not for long. Using DDT to protect crops had made the local *Anopheles* species resistant. Widespread malaria set in again, with *falciparum* appearing for the first time.

The WHO thereafter switched gears from the lofty goal of eradication to the drudgery of control. Changing priorities took time. Experts were in short supply. For years no one had wanted to study a disease assumed to be doomed to extinction. As one biologist put it, the global eradication campaign didn't get rid of malaria, but it got rid of malariologists.

Eventually, the WHO turned back to the tried-and-true, to draining swamps and killing larvae, hanging up screens and passing out mosquito nets.

Though often criticized as a failure, the eradication campaign achieved some triumphs. Eleven nations—five in the Caribbean, four in Europe, plus Chile and Taiwan—had indeed eliminated malaria. In the late 1960s the Netherlands became the last northern European country to do so. Cuba followed a few years later. Follow-up efforts over the next three decades pushed the disease out of much of northern and central Asia, roughly half its range in South America, and virtually every shore touched by the Mediterranean Sea.

Even in areas where malaria returned, it was often less severe than in the past. The campaign had also trained local experts in public health strategies—an ongoing benefit to developing countries. Anti-malaria efforts introduced the developing world to chloroquine. If the drug was less effective in some places, it remained useful elsewhere for years. During its heyday, it allowed millions of people sufficient good health to better their lives or a chance to grow up without the threat of death or disability.

But it was hard to overlook the implications of the failed campaign and the devastating setbacks caused by drug resistance. The magic bullet, available for ten or fifteen cents a dose, was becoming more and more worthless against the deadliest parasite. In fact, it had transformed *falciparum* into one of the first recognized iatrogenic illnesses—diseases that evolved in reaction to medical treatment. In Southeast Asia, it took the parasite only a few years to start to shake off the replacement drug, Fansidar (pyrimethanine-sulfadoxine). The next generation of drugs failed even more quickly.

Despite enormous effort and the best intentions, one of humanity's greatest killers had survived, harder to treat than ever. And it was spreading.

five
Disease of
the Poor

At least 300 million people worldwide suffer from malaria symptoms every year. Between 1 and 3 million of them die, the great majority African children under age five.

To live in sub-Saharan Africa is to live with malaria. The problems it causes were so profound the WHO never attempted to implement its eradication program in the region. Because malaria and humans evolved together in Africa, the disease is hyperadapted to thrive in many local environments. All the factors that encourage malaria transmission exist. All are intensified by both nature and human activity.

Climate plays a huge role. In the northern countries that cleared malaria, the disease was mostly a seasonal problem confined to the summer. But Africa's tropical rains and heat create ideal breeding conditions for both parasites and mosquitoes year-round.

A doctor cradles the head of a child infected with malaria in Uganda, in east Africa. *(Courtesy of John Stanmeyer/VII/AP Images)*

Warm weather has a measurable effect on mosquito breeding. The time the eggs need to hatch in the mosquito's stomach decreases in higher temperatures. That makes it more likely the infected insect will live long enough to pass on the disease. Research also shows that if the temperature increases from sixty-six degrees Fahrenheit to seventy degrees, females of certain species take blood meals every three days instead of every four. Over a month's time that translates to about two more feedings per mosquito multiplied by tens of thousands of mosquitoes. More infected bites means more malaria. More uninfected bites increases the chances a mosquito without parasites will draw some into its body. That in turn increases the potential for infected bites.

Then there's the mosquito itself. Most sub-Saharan Africans catch their malaria from *Anopheles gambiae*. Exposure to *Homo sapiens* since prehistory and the related evolutionary pressures have closely tied *A. gambiae* to malaria. The species' behaviors powerfully amplify its power to pass on disease.

Where the several *Anopheles* species in the U.S. or India would as soon feed on livestock or other animals, *A. gambiae* bites human beings over 90 percent of the time. It's also an opportunistic breeder. *A. gambiae* will lay its eggs in water in hoofprints or discarded plastic jugs or the holes created when villagers cut mud bricks to build homes. Adding to the problem is the fact *A. gambiae* lives longer than many *Anopheles* species. Longevity allows an infected *A. gambiae* mosquito to bite, breed, and transmit malaria more often than, say, the major American or Indian vectors.

Malariologists consider a vector's longevity an important part of the malaria problem. It figures into the basic reproduction number (BRN) that scientists use to measure a disease's

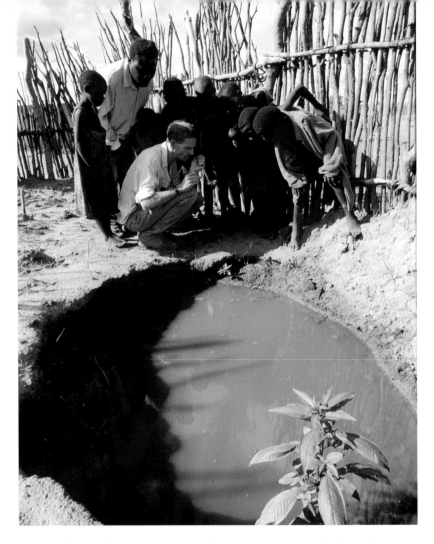

Children in Zimbabwe, in southern Africa, examine a pool of standing water as they are taught about the life cycle of mosquitoes and the dangers of malaria. *(Courtesy of Neil Cooper/Alamy)*

power to transmit itself. In general, a BRN of two means an infected individual will pass the disease on to two other people. Smallpox, for example, has a BRN in the three-to-five range, depending on circumstances. It is considered a contagious disease. By comparison, malaria's BRN can zoom to more than one hundred in a situation where *A. gambiae* is the main vector.

But the unlucky hand dealt by nature doesn't fully explain why a well-understood and easy-to-treat disease continues to afflict millions of Africans or, for that matter, millions of Brazilians, Indians, and Papua New Guineans. The reason is poverty.

Not all poor countries have malaria. But all malarial countries have huge numbers of poor people. And most of the world's very poorest countries are in sub-Saharan Africa. As was the case in Sardinia or the Tennessee Valley, poverty encourages malaria to thrive. At the same time, malaria drains resources and human potential to such an extent that it contributes to self-perpetuating poverty.

Poor countries as a rule lack the money to spend on public health services. Not surprisingly, most sub-Saharan Africans do not have access to the most basic health care.

Malaria strikes rural areas hardest. It's there where people have the fewest resources and are most at the mercy of the kind of everyday health hazards like malnutrition and poor drinking water that leave people vulnerable to disease. It's also the landscape preferred by mosquitoes.

A rural African with malaria has few options. A poor country's infrastructure—or lack of it—works in every way against getting proper treatment. Roads are bad and vehicles few. If the patient somehow gets to a clinic, it often lacks electricity. In all likelihood no doctors or nurses work there. The region is short of both, short of the schools to turn out more, short of teachers to staff schools. Or, the government pays health care workers so little that many of them move to richer countries to make a living. Even facilities with full-time staff seldom have the equipment needed to effectively treat malaria. A diagnosis may be wrong because the doctors lack the microscopes needed to spot parasites in blood.

The medicines used add to the problem. Chloroquine and Fansidar are the only widely available drugs. Neither works well anymore. Lariam (mefloquine), the antimalarial of choice in the U.S., costs too much and is hard to find in much of Africa.

If a victim somehow gets medicine to clear the parasites, it only means short-term relief. In heavily malarial areas a person gets bitten by infected mosquitoes three times a night. The sheer numbers of insects is mind-boggling. According to research, Africans in the hardest-hit areas would have to wipe out half the living *A. gambiae* every day *for five consecutive years* to make a dent in the transmission cycle.

Malaria also takes a heavy economic toll. The WHO's figures show a heavily malarial country loses a fifth of its economic strength every fifteen years. Other studies suggest that malaria costs the continent an estimated $12 billion every year. Countries hit hardest must spend around 40 percent of their inadequate health care budgets on this single disease at the expense of other serious problems.

The effects reverberate across the entire economy. As used to happen in the American South, malaria keeps workers from working. A bout of malaria costs a worker between four and six days on the job. Recovery takes four to eight more days. Those able to recuperate on their feet get less done due to weakness. Those with the types of malaria that lingers in the body for years—and West Africa hosts all three—simply never feel well.

In agricultural areas, a malaria epidemic has terrible effects if it strikes during the harvest. Most farmers in sub-Saharan Africa practice subsistence farming. What they grow is what they have to eat. Since most African farmers barely grow enough to live on in the best years, a case of fever at harvest time means less food gets picked. That can lead to nutritional problems or starvation, not just for the farmer but for his extended family.

On a countrywide scale, malaria damages what economists call *human capital*. Human capital consists of the skills and ability to work that citizens put into their nation's economies. It is improved by making workers healthier, better trained, and better educated. Malaria acts as a drag on all those aspects of society. For example, malaria can cause lifelong neurological damage that often leads to learning disabilities or, in the worst cases, to mental retardation. It keeps children out of school on a regular basis, and makes it hard to learn or work during the time it takes to get better.

A lack of human capital in turn discourages outsiders from investing in a country. No company wants to build a factory or start a mining operation with a workforce that's too sick to show up part of the time. Poor education damages the potential for more advanced industries. No investment means no jobs, certainly no jobs at good wages. Governments thus miss out on the tax revenues needed to build hospitals or improve the infrastructure necessary to facilitate a strong economy, such as roads and water treatment. Nor can trade take root. Merchants are leery of investing or visiting. The same goes for tourism, a potentially profitable industry. Africa offers breathtaking scenery, but many people won't risk malaria to see it.

Everyone agrees pushing back malaria will take a lot of money. Anne Mills, a health economist at the London School of Hygiene and Tropical medicine, says, "[Malaria] control will not make much progress unless the international community is willing to tackle the gross underfunding and major problems of health-service infrastructure in Africa."

According to Harvard economist Jeffrey Sachs, "Extreme poverty can be cut sharply in a decade's time by scaling up investments in key infrastructure (such as roads, power, water, and sanitation) and human capital (such as education, nutrition, health care, and family planning). Such investments would not only improve living conditions [in ten years], but would help the poorest countries to achieved sustained economic growth after that date."

Few doubt that economic development would help Africans, or for that matter people in other malarial regions. It's sadly ironic, then, that development can, in the short term, make malaria worse because it changes the environment.

Brazil, for instance, has spent the last generation developing the Amazon rain forest region. Environmental degradation continues to be rife, however, with deforestation a leading problem.

Brazilian farmers cut trees for slash-and-burn agriculture. When they move on, they leave behind them shrubby landscapes preferred by the malaria vector, *Anopheles darlingi*. One recent study claims *A. darlingi* bites far more often in areas where a quarter to a third of the forest is cut. Conditions in the rain forest are so ideal that the species is out-breeding other mosquitoes for supremacy in the new habitat. As a result, malaria is an ongoing crisis.

New mines are another contributor to the problem. In a rain forest climate, water continually collects in the holes that are an inevitable part of a mining operation. Mosquitoes then breed in the water. To aggravate the problem, settlers from

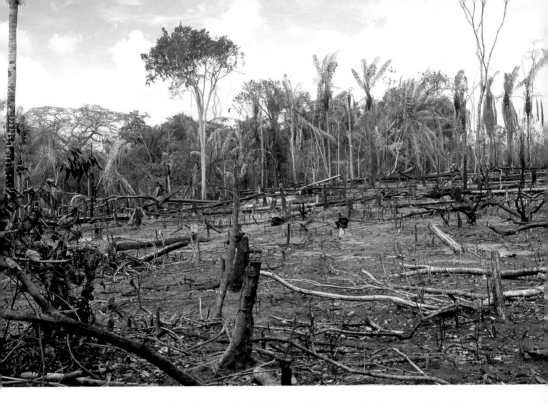

A photo depicting the aftermath of slash-and-burn agriculture used to clear a Brazilian rain forest. Such farming methods create ideal conditions for malaria mosquitoes to breed. *(Courtesy of Worldwide Picture Library/Alamy)*

Brazil's coast migrated to the Amazonian frontier and ran into unfamiliar types of jungle malaria. Use of antimalarial drugs soared, pressuring the parasites to evolve resistance.

Despite such aftershocks, however, economic development remains a vital part of malaria control. The goal is to find a balance between economic needs and public health matters. By now it's clear that ignoring nature usually boomerangs on human beings.

Not all the news is bad. Programs to alleviate malaria have picked up in recent years, thanks to scientific advances, new sources of money, and a renewed interest in tropical diseases. One of the most promising breakthroughs has been a new antimalarial drug.

In the 1960s, China's government embarked on a program to develop medicines and other products from Chinese sources. Researchers dug through the country's long tradition of herbal remedies and folk medicine looking for cures. During the search, they discovered that the ancients used qinghao—the sweet wormwood plant—for malaria. Chinese scientists eventually isolated the antimalarial agent, qinghaosu, called in the West artemisinin. Tests showed that artemisinin cleared parasites from the bloodstream much faster than quinine-based drugs like chloroquine. In particular it knocked out *falciparum* before a massive build-up of parasites brought on deadly cerebral malaria.

Artemisinin was ignored outside Asia until the early 1980s. The West relied instead on mefloquine, the newest drug derived from quinine. Marketed widely as Larium, mefloquine did a good job of preventing malaria. It was also very expensive compared to chloroquine.

In 1981, American malariologist Kyle Webster and British colleagues traveled to China to meet researchers in that country. Two professors gave the visitors a bottle of powdered artemisinin compound. Some time later Webster was working in Thailand and caught one of the region's strains of multi-drug-resistant malaria. A Thai colleague working with the artemisinin gave Webster an experimental medicine.

Webster went in to work the next day. In a week the drug had cleared the parasites from his body.

News began to spread. Unfortunately, so did malaria able to resist multiple drugs, particularly in Thailand's border regions. Mefloquine, though fairly new, was no longer 100 percent reliable.

The Chinese released an artemisinin-based drug, artesunate, for oral use. (There was also a related drug for injections called artemether.) The WHO initially downplayed artesunate. When it became clear the parasites had figured out mefloquine, however, the organization took another look.

Experts knew that, used alone, artesunate might pressure parasites into evolving resistance. That would be a disaster, since it was the last totally effective antimalarial drug. Ominously, artemisinin-based drugs like artesunate were already being used and misused in Southeast Asia—in other words, in one of the places where chloroquine resistance developed, and in all likelihood the source of the drug-resistant malaria burning its way across Africa.

If use was a problem, abuse threatened to cause a crisis. For instance, the gem hunters along Thai's border regions often couldn't find pure artesunate and instead took weak or counterfeit versions. Malaria experts working in Thailand's border regions recently found that the local fakes contained traces of artemisinin to fool tests. Such weakened drugs can't kill *falciparum*. Instead, it exposes the parasite to just enough of the drug to encourage adaptation and resistance, in much the same way the overuse of chloroquine did in the 1950s and 1960s.

To head off drug resistance, researchers combined artesunate with existing drugs. These artemisinin-based combination therapies, or ACTs, hit the parasites in two different ways. Those not killed by one drug fell to the other. Partnering with artesunate also seemed to restore mefloquine's potency, an unexpected bonus.

Still, uncertainties lingered about side effects. ACTs remain unapproved by the U.S. government. And there's the resistance problem. Asians can still buy straight artesunate and related drugs. Similar medications filter into Africa.

In 2006, the WHO raised the alarm. "It is critical that artemisinins be used correctly," said Dr. Lee Jong-wook, the WHO director-general. "We request pharmaceutical companies to immediately stop marketing single-drug artemisinin tablets and instead market [ACTs] only."

With the WHO and other aid groups advocating ACTs, African countries have begun to embrace the new drugs. Kenya, with 34,000 child deaths a year, recently promised to spend $21 million on the new drugs and train health workers in its use. In neighboring Uganda, a local corporation plans to make an ACT using sweet wormwood grown by local farmers.

An ACT dose can sell for about $1.50 (about forty cents for a child's dose). But that's still a lot of money for the average African, particularly because it's necessary to buy multiple doses of artemisinin-based drugs to get well. At present, making ACTs available to Africans will take at least $2 billion for ACT doses alone, and that's a conservative estimate. According to Doctors Without Borders, seven of every ten countries that have promised to adopt ACTs continue to use chloroquine or related medicines because of financial problems, lack of education and health workers, and ACT shortages.

The high cost of separating artemisinin from sweet wormwood inflates the drug's price. Reduce that cost, the price comes down. University of California Berkeley researchers may be on the way to doing just that. A team announced in 2006 that it had bio-engineered yeast able to turn a related compound into artemisinic acid. If perfected, the process could eliminate the need for sweet wormwood and cut the drug's price to something closer to that of chloroquine.

Unless and until that happens, however, funding remains *the* issue. The need to use every dollar wisely has inspired a variety of low-tech suggestions. As drug advocates learned the lesson about evolving parasites, so these experts keep environmental concerns in mind. Among the ideas:

- Stocking lakes and ponds with the larvae-eating Gambusia fish, as in Italy and Spain.
- Mixing cow dung into small mosquito breeding pools, in those areas where mosquitoes breed in small pools and where people have cows.
- Passing out sweet wormwood seeds so people can grow their own plants and make their own malaria-fighting tea.

Without a doubt, however, insecticide-treated bed nets are the low-tech idea of the moment.

Treated nets are a centerpiece of the WHO's Roll Back Malaria initiative. Started in 1998, Roll Back Malaria works with UNICEF, the World Bank, and other global agencies toward the declared goal of cutting malaria cases in half. Roll Back Malaria coordinates control and education efforts through partnerships with affected countries, development groups, researchers, private companies, and charitable foundations.

If used right, the nets get results—studies show that deaths in children under five drop dramatically. One Tanzanian village used as a model reported zero malaria a year after each of its 167 people received a free net.

The tightly-woven nets cover sleeping areas. Nets can be treated with long-lasting insecticide that paralyzes mosquitoes on contact. Until recently, the net needed to be

A worker at a Tanzanian company that produces insecticidal bed nets. *(Courtesy of Charles Ommanney/ Getty Images)*

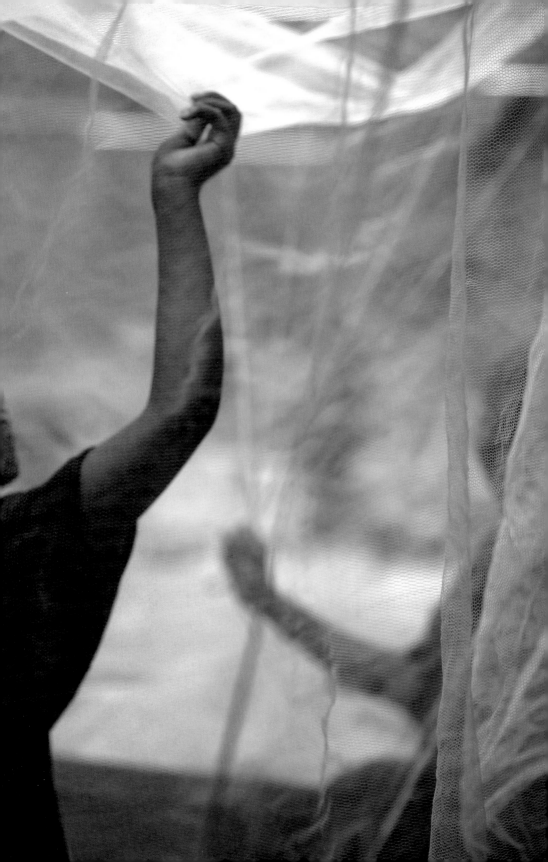

dipped in insecticide to recharge its power against mosquitoes. The chemical on newer-generation nets lasts up to five years.

At a price of two to ten dollars per net, however, bed nets remain out of reach for most Africans. Aid groups therefore buy nets to give away. Roll Back Malaria and a number of partners, including various Red Cross organizations, handed out 2 million nets in Niger in late 2005 and early 2006. Mothers received one free after vaccinating their children for polio. Bed-net programs aim in particular at preschool children, the group most vulnerable to death or disability. The idea is to protect children until age five—the insecticide remains potent for that long for a reason. Statistics show the chance of survival increases from that age on.

Bed nets have limits. Tropical heat further discourages some Africans from using them. A net that keeps out mosquitoes also keeps out a cooling breeze. In addition, not everyone believes they work. A number of people blame malaria on the sun or bad food. Even those who buy into nets, and who use them correctly, can still be bitten while outdoors. Getting people to use them the right way presents its own set of problems. Officials in Namibia recently pleaded with men not to use the nets for fishing.

The difficult circumstances in Africa and elsewhere have led some to suggest a controversial solution: bringing back DDT.

Despite the American ban, DDT has continued to be used in a few nations. In fact, it's manufactured today in India and remains an important part of its malaria-control program.

Experts aren't surprised. "There is no practical replacement for DDT, nor is there likely to be in 2007, 2017, or 2027,"

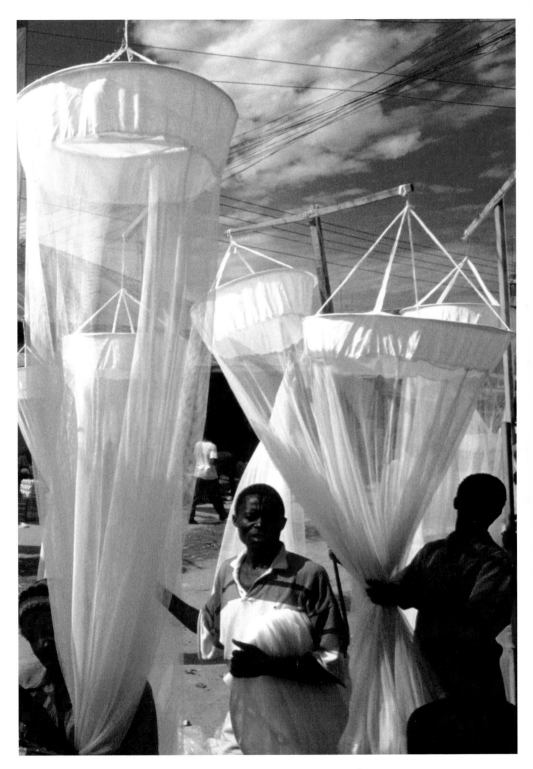

Mosquito nets for sale at a market in Tanzania, in east Africa. *(Courtesy of Eye Ubiquitous/Alamy)*

wrote malariologist Robert S. Desowitz. "When a poor tropical country runs into epidemic malaria trouble, they have no recourse but to resort to DDT household spraying to save their citizens."

DDT's low cost increases the temptation to use it. Using expensive alternative pesticides—some of them costing five times as much as DDT—drains budgets. Mosquitoes can adapt to replacement insecticides, too. Some mosquitoes in India, for example, resist not only DDT but its first, second, and third alternatives.

The same problem troubles South Africa in areas bordering heavily malarial Mozambique, among the world's poorest countries. A boom in South African cotton farming brought on an increased use of insecticides. The chemicals ran off into water sources where mosquitoes bred, encouraging resistance. A sudden outbreak of malaria in 2000 left the South Africans without an effective weapon against mosquitoes. Public health officials turned to DDT. Ever since, a program of indoor spraying and drug therapy has reduced cases from 45,000 per year to less than 1,500.

Advocates argue that the South African example prove it's time to remove the stigma from DDT. Environmental groups disagree, citing the chemical's well-documented effects on animal life. A year after the South African outbreak, several leading groups persuaded more than ninety countries to sign the Stockholm Convention on Persistent Organic Pollutants. The international treaty included language to eliminate DDT worldwide.

After malaria experts mounted a protest, the agreement was altered to allow for indoor spraying under certain circumstances that met a tough set of rules.

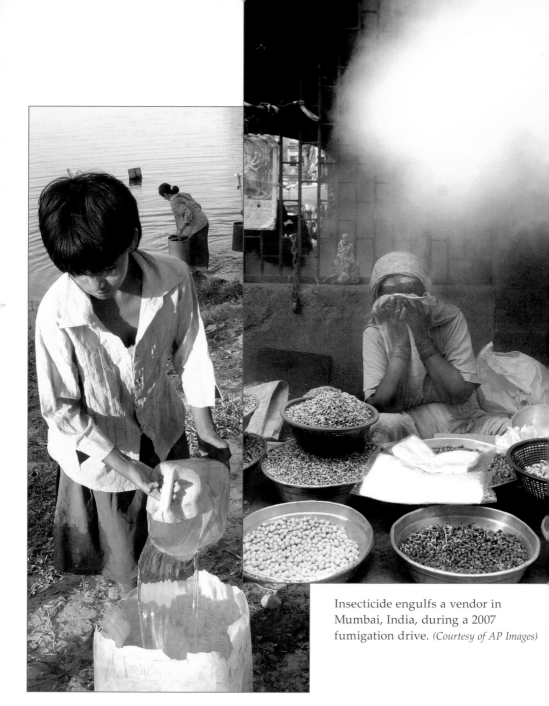

Insecticide engulfs a vendor in Mumbai, India, during a 2007 fumigation drive. *(Courtesy of AP Images)*

A girl pours water as villagers in the background collect their own from a lake near a village in Myanmar, a country hit hard by malaria. *(Courtesy of Khin Maung Win/AFP/Getty Images)*

Some environmentalists concede the occasional need to use the chemical, while stating that a future ban is still preferable. Nonetheless, the U.S. and European governments resisted change. African nations, needing trade partners, and fearing threats to cut off aid money if they used DDT, went along. When Uganda announced plans to use the chemical for malaria control, the European Union warned of possible negative effects on the country's produce and plant exports.

Opinion may be shifting, though. In early 2006, the Union added that nothing would happen if Uganda obeyed the Stockholm treaty rules. Around the same time, the U.S. promised $20 million for indoor spraying in eight countries. Three of them intend to use DDT, with the U.S. government's blessing.

Should DDT come back, it may be possible to cut the risks by pinpointing where it's needed. Climatologists have developed models to predict the weather patterns known to drive malaria epidemics. Reliable forecasts would allow authorities to rush supplies—whether medicine, nets, or insecticides—to areas before an outbreak, rather than reacting to it afterward.

Low-tech approaches to malaria continue to play the leading role in campaigns against the disease. But recent scientific advances have brought attention to high-tech research taking place in biotechnology and a number of other fields. The future of malaria control may be built on scientific work being done in labs today.

Of all the current directions being explored, a malaria vaccine gets the most attention. Vaccines have been successful against other diseases. A vaccine made it possible to eradicate smallpox—one of the greatest public health triumphs of the last century. Ideally, a vaccine offers lifelong (or at least long-

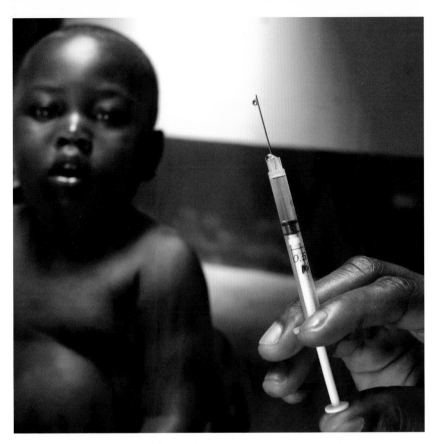

A child looks at a needle prior to receiving a vaccination in Ghana, Africa in 2007. Although vaccines have had success in eradicating other diseases, scientists have yet to develop a vaccine against a parasite. *(Courtesy of Shaul Schwarz/Getty Images)*

time) immunity. In malaria's case, a vaccine would have the added benefit of liberating those in malarial countries from toxic drugs and insecticide pollution.

The problem is, no one has ever developed a vaccine against a parasite. Thus far humanity's successes have come against viruses, like smallpox, and disease-causing bacteria, like diphtheria. *Plasmodium falciparum* and the other malaria parasites are microscopic animals. As such, they're more genetically complex. The polio virus, for example, has a handful of genes. A malaria parasite has around 5,000, making it a much harder target.

The apparent success of chloroquine and DDT ended vaccine research almost before it started. Interest in a malaria vaccine only revived after the eradication campaign failed. It took time to get up to speed. Then scandal dogged the field for years. Two scientists in two different cases ended up facing charges for steering research funds aside for personal use. In another case, a U.S. government official in charge of vaccine money was named as part of a plot to cash in through filing false tax returns and smuggling monkeys.

Even the legal activities have been controversial. Feuds have erupted over funding and experiment results. Officials handing out money often had little background in malaria and ignored experts' advice. Test vaccines failed, or had limited results, or were too dangerous to try out on humans.

For-profit corporations lead the way in the Western nations when it comes to developing, manufacturing, and distributing medicine. Because vaccines don't make money, companies have no incentive to invest in research. To encourage vaccine development, nonprofit entities have allied with drug companies. The nonprofits donate research money and promise to buy working vaccines in bulk. The drug companies provide the know-how and manufacturing.

In 2004, a partnership between the Bill and Melinda Gates Foundation through the pharmaceutical company GlaxoSmithKline led to vaccine tests in Mozambique. The vaccine combined a piece of the *falciparum* sporozoite—the phase of the parasite injected by a mosquito—with a piece of hepatitis B, a virus known to provoke a strong immune response in humans. If it worked, the vaccine would provoke an immune response able to wipe out or reduce the number of parasitic invaders before they reached the liver to reproduce. Results showed the vaccine cut the risk by 57 percent of *falciparum* in children aged one to four. In children under two the rate was a hopeful 77 percent.

Poverty, however, dampens even the promise of vaccines. Should the Mozambique vaccine pass the approval process, for example, its price—somewhere between $10 and $20 per dose—means richer nations will have to pay for any large-scale vaccination program. Even then, there's still no guarantee a vaccine would get to the Africans who need it. Reasonably cheap and safe vaccines for measles and other childhood diseases reach at best half the children in sub-Saharan Africa. In some places it's much less. Events like wars, government instability, and natural disasters often interrupt the programs that get off the ground.

The high-tech solutions don't stop at vaccines. Scientists have recently started to look at genetic engineering.

In 2002, researchers announced they had mapped the *falciparum* genome. In the short term, understanding the parasite on a genetic level may reveal weaknesses in its structure that a vaccine can exploit. Down the road, it may be possible to engineer a new *Anopheles* mosquito—one unable to carry malaria parasites. The hope is that an engineered mosquito can out-compete nature's species in the wild and eventually replace malaria-carrying insects. To say the least, engineered mosquitoes present a long list of questions, not least of which is how they will behave or mutate once in the ecosystem. Chloroquine and DDT are both reminders of the dangers of tinkering with nature.

Such solutions, if possible, are years and maybe decades in the future. There are critics who wonder why malaria's limited research funds get spent on uncertain and expensive high-tech projects. Said Robert Gwadz of the U.S. National Institute of Allergy and Infectious Diseases, "Where malaria has been controlled anywhere in the world, it has been done by controlling mosquitoes, not through vaccines or genetics or anything fancy."

Limited money, widespread poverty, an adaptable adversary, disagreements over solutions—it is easy to look at the malaria problem and feel hopeless. But there is reason for hope. Programs like Roll Back Malaria represent, if nothing else, an effort to raise awareness of malaria and its effects on societies in the developing world. The tremendous amounts of money handed out by the Gates Foundation has expanded existing efforts into new areas and revived old research and public health programs that a few years ago looked finished for good. Lower-profile efforts—whether distributing ACTs and bed nets or conducting high-tech research—contribute already.

In recent years a number of new groups have been founded. The Global Fund to Fight AIDS, Tuberculosis, and Malaria acts as a clearinghouse for donor money and supports on-the-ground distribution of bed nets and other similar plans. Instead of implementing programs itself, the Fund reviews and chooses programs based in needy countries and commits grant money to those it believes have the greatest chance to make progress.

The Malaria Vaccine Initiative, begun in 1999, aims at vaccine development. Working with the Program for Appropriate Technology in Health (PATH), the MVI draws together corporations, governments, and researchers, and at the same time helps coordinate vaccine tests in Africa and elsewhere.

Medicines for Malaria was set up in 1999 and backed by foundations, the United Nations, and governments with up to

$30 million per year. The goal: to support research for a new set of anti-malaria drugs every five years.

Malaria's current range is vast, but not as wide as a century ago. Then, few considered it possible to drive the disease from Italy or the shores of North Africa, places endemic since ancient times. The eradication campaign, though widely considered a failure or lost opportunity, can still be a stepping stone to something better. Every day research continues and knowledge advances. Amidst all the possibilities, one thing is certain. If the effort against malaria is going to succeed, it will have to be as relentless as malaria itself.

Sources

INTRODUCTION

p. 11-12, "There is no aspect . . ." Berton Roueche, *The Medical Detectives, Volume II* (New York: Dutton, 1984), 223.

p. 12, "He had a fever . . ." William Shakespeare, *The Tragedy of Julius Caesar* (New York: Washington Square Press, 1959).

CHAPTER TWO: The Roman Disease

p. 23, "In the area . . ." William H. McNeill, *Plagues and Peoples* (Garden City, NY: Anchor Press/Doubleday, 1976), 88.

p. 24, "[F]or whenever the great heat . . ." Roy Porter, *The Greatest Benefit to Mankind* (New York: W. W. Norton & Company, 1997), 60.

p. 24, "The least dangerous . . ." Roueche, *The Medical Detectives, V. II*, 217.

p. 26-27, "Precautions should . . . be taken . . ." John Scarborough, *Roman Medicine* (Ithaca, NY: Cornell University Press, 1969), 81.

p. 27, "What can I do . . ." Ibid.

p. 33, "numerous illness that . . ." A. Roger Ekrich, *At Day's Close: Night in Times Past* (New York: W. W. Norton, 2005), 13.

p. 33, "Tremble and go . . ." Roueche, *The Medical Detectives , V. II,* 218.

p. 37, "Our men were destroyed . . ." James Horn, *A Land as God Made It* (New York: Basic Books, 2005), 57.

p. 38, "thrice worse than Essex . . ." Carl Bridenbaugh, *Jamestown: 1544-1699* (New York: Oxford University Press, 1980), 47.

p. 38, "They who want . . ." Fiammetta Rocco, *The Miraculous Fever Tree* (New York: HarperCollins, 2003), 174.

CHAPTER THREE: The Fever Tree and the Magic Bullet

p. 47, "America is rich . . ." Mark Honigsbaum, *The Fever Trail: In Search of the Cure for Malaria* (New York: Farrar, Straus, and Giroux, 2001), 51.

p. 55, "Malarial fever . . . haunts " Porter, *The Greatest Benefit to Mankind,* 465.

p. 57, "Intermittent fever is . . ." Roueche, *The Medical Detectives, V. II,* 219.

p. 58, "I was astonished . . ." Robert S. Desowitz, *The Malaria Capers* (New York: W. W. Norton, 1991), 167.

p. 64, "Those were trying times . . ." Library of Congress American Life Histories, interview with Mrs. Mary Bickett.

p. 66, "for the South . . ." Robert S. Desowitz, *Who Gave Pinta to the Santa Maria?* (New York: W. W. Norton, 1997), 195.

p. 66, "I suffered with malaria . . ." Library of Congress American Life Histories, interview with Martin Cross.

p. 68, "This will be . . ." Honigsbaum, *The Fever Trail,* 210.

CHAPTER FOUR: Eradication

p. 72, "the most important addition . . ." Gordon Harrison, *Mosquitoes, Malaria, and Man: A History of the Hostilities Since 1880* (New York: E. P. Dutton, 1978), 187.

p. 72-73, "[T]he distribution of quinine . . ." Darwin H. Stapleton, "Lessons of History? Anti-malarial strategies of the International Health Board and the Rockefeller Foundation from the 1920s to the era of DDT," *Public Health Reports* 29 (March-April 2004): 209.

p. 76, "After the DDT solution . . ." G. Fischer, "Presentation speech for the Nobel Prize in Physiology or Medicine, 1948."

p. 76, "The locals regarded this . . ." Malcolm Gladwell, "The mosquito killer," *New Yorker*, July 2, 2001, 46.

p. 82, "There is . . . reason to fear," World Health Organization, "The World Health Organization and malaria eradication," World Health Organization report WHO/Mal/162, February 1, 1956.

p. 83, "[I]f countries . . ." *The Coming Plague: Newly Emerging Diseases in a World Out of Balance* (New York: Penguin, 1994), 48.

p. 87, "It's all over . . ." Ibid., 50.

p. 93, "The world has heard much . . ." Rachel Carson, *Silent Spring* (Boston, MA: Houghton Mifflin, 1962), 266.

p. 94, "Practical advice should be . . ." Ibid., 275.

CHAPTER FIVE: Disease of the Poor

p. 103-104, "[Malaria] control will not . . ." Declan Butler, "What difference does a genome make?," *Nature,* October 3, 2002, 428.

p. 104, "Extreme poverty can be cut . . ." Jeffrey D.
Sachs, "Achieving the Millennium Development Goals—
The case for malaria," *New England Journal of Medicine*,
January 13, 2005, 115.

p. 108, "It is critical . . ." World Health Organization, "WHO
calls for an immediate halt to provision of single-drug
artemisinin malaria pills," press release, January 19, 2006.

p. 112-113, "There is no practical replacement . . ." Robert S.
Desowitz, *Federal Bodysnatchers and the New Guinea
Virus* (New York: W. W. Norton, 2002), 73.

p. 120, "Where malaria has been controlled . . ." Gretchen
Vogel, "In pursuit of a killer," *Science* 298, no. 5591
(October 4, 2002): 87.

Bibliography

BOOKS

Arrian, Aubrey De Sélincourt, trans. *The Campaigns of Alexander.* New York: Penguin, 1971.

Atchity, Kenneth J., ed. *The Classical Greek Reader.* New York: Henry Holt, 1998.

Bridenbaugh, Carl. *Jamestown: 1544–1699.* New York: Oxford University Press, 1980.

Burnet, Macfarlane, and David O. White. *Natural History of Infectious Disease.* Cambridge: Cambridge University Press, 1972.

Carpopino, Jérôme, and Henry T. Rowell, eds. *Daily Life in Ancient Rome.* Translated by E. O. Lorimer. New Haven, CT: Yale University Press, 1968.

Carson, Rachel. *Silent Spring.* Boston, MA: Houghton Mifflin, 1962.

Crosby, Albert W., Jr. *The Columbian Exchange.* Westport, CT: Greenwood Press, 1972.

DeSalle, Rob, ed. *Epidemic: The World of Infectious Disease.* New York: Free Press, 1999.

Desowitz, Robert S. *Federal Bodysnatchers and the New Guinea Virus.* New York: W. W. Norton, 2002.

———. *The Malaria Capers.* New York: W. W. Norton, 1991.

———. *Who Gave Pinta to the Santa Maria?* New York: W. W. Norton, 1997.

Diamond, Jared. *Guns, Germs, and Steel.* New York: W. W. Norton, 1999.

Ehrlich, Paul and Anne. *Extinction: The Causes and Consequences of the Disappearance of Species.* New York: Random House, 1981.

Ekrich, A. Roger. *At Day's Close: Night in Times Past.* New York: W. W. Norton, 2005.

Frank, Richard B. *Guadalcanal.* New York: Random House, 1990.

Friedrich, Otto. *The End of the World: A History.* New York: Fromm, 1994.

Galen. *Selected Works.* Translated by P. N. Singer. New York: Oxford University Press, 1997.

Garrett, Laurie. *Betrayal of Trust: The Collapse of Global Public Health.* New York: Hyperion, 2000.

———. *The Coming Plague: Newly Emerging Diseases in a World Out of Balance.* New York: Penguin Books, 1994.

Green, Peter. *Alexander of Macedon, 356–323 B.C.: A Historical Biography.* Berkeley, CA: University of California Press, 1991.

———. *Armada from Athens.* New York: Doubleday and Co., 1970.

Harrison, Gordon. *Mosquitoes, Malaria, and Man: A History of the Hostilities Since 1880.* New York: E. P. Dutton, 1978.

Hobhouse, Henry. *Seeds of Change: Five Plants that Transformed Mankind.* New York: Harper & Row, 1986.

Honigsbaum, Mark. *The Fever Trail: In Search of the Cure for Malaria.* New York: Farrar, Straus, and Giroux, 2001.

Horn, James. *A Land as God Made It.* New York: Basic Books, 2005.

Hudson, Charles. *The Southeastern Indians.* Knoxville, TN: University of Tennessee Press, 1976.

Von Humboldt, Alexander, and Thomasina Ross, eds. and trans. *Personal Narrative of Travels to the Equinoctial Regions of American during the Years 1799–1804, Volume 1.* London: George Bell and Sons, 1889.

Karlen, Arno. *Man and Microbes.* New York: G. P. Putnam's Sons, 1995.

Major, Ralph H., M.D. *Fatal Partners: War and Disease.* Garden City, NY: Doubleday, Doren, and Co., 1941.

Mann, Charles. *1491: New Revelations of the Americas Before Columbus.* New York: Knopf, 2005.

Mayor, Adrienne. *Greek Fire, Poison Arrows, and Scorpion Bombs.* Woodstock, NY: Overlook Duckworth, 2003.

McCullough, David. *The Path Between the Seas.* New York: Simon and Schuster, 1974.

McNeill, William H. *Plagues and Peoples.* Garden City, NY: Anchor Press/Doubleday, 1976.

Mintz, Sidney W. *Sweetness and Power: The Place of Sugar in Modern History.* New York: Viking Penguin, 1985.

Moorehead, Alan. *The White Nile.* New York: Harper & Row, 1971.

Morales, Waltraud Q. *A Brief History of Bolivia.* New York: Facts on File, 2003.

Morgan, Ted. *Wilderness at Dawn: The Settling of the North American Continent.* New York: Simon and Schuster, 1993.

Nikiforuk, Andrew. *The Fourth Horseman.* New York: M. Evans & Company, 1991.

Porter, Roy. *The Greatest Benefit to Mankind.* New York: W. W. Norton & Company, 1997.

Rocco, Fiammetta. *The Miraculous Fever Tree: Malaria and the Quest for a Cure that Changed the World.* New York: HarperCollins, 2003.

Roueche, Berton. *The Medical Detectives, Volume II.* New York: Dutton, 1984.

Sachs, Jeffrey D. *The End of Poverty.* New York: Penguin, 2005.

Scarborough, John. *Roman Medicine.* Ithaca, NY: Cornell University Press, 1969.

Shakespeare, William. *The Tragedy of Julius Caesar.* New York: Washington Square Press, 1959.

Sheehan, Bernard W. *Savagism and Civility: Indians and Englishmen in Colonial Virginia.* Cambridge: Cambridge University Press, 1980.

Spielman, Andrew, and Michael D'Antonio. *Mosquito: A Natural History of Our Most Persistent and Deadly Foe.* New York: Hyperion, 2001.

Stannard, David E. *American Holocaust: The Conquest of the New World.* New York: Oxford University Press, 1992.

Suetonius, Robert Graves, trans. *The Twelve Caesars.* Edited by Michael Grant. New York: Viking Penguin, 1984.

Thomas, Hugh. *The Slave Trade.* New York: Simon and Schuster, 1997.

Thucydides. *The Peloponnesian War.* Translated by T. E. Wick. New York: Modern Library, 1982.

Vlekke, Bernard H. M. *The Story of the Dutch East Indies.* Cambridge, MA: Harvard University Press, 1945.

White, John Manchip. *Cortés and the Downfall of the Aztec Empire.* New York: Carroll & Graf, 1996.

Wilson, James. *The Earth Shall Weep: A History of Native America.* New York: Atlantic Monthly Press, 1998.

NEWSPAPERS AND PERIODICALS

Arrow, Kenneth J., Hellen Gelband, and Dean T. Jamison. "Making antimalarial agents available in Africa." *New England Journal of Medicine* (July 28, 2005): 333–35.

Baird, J. Kevin. "Effectiveness of antimalarial drugs." *New England Journal of Medicine* 352, no. 15 (April 14, 2005): 1565–77.

Budiansky, Stephen. "Creatures of our own making." *Science* 298, no. 5591 (October 4, 2002): 80–86.

Butler, Declan. "What difference does a genome make?" *Nature* 419, no. 6906 (Octobert 3, 2002): 426–28.

Clarke, Tom. "Mosquitoes minus malaria." *Nature* 419, no. 690 (Oct. 3, 2002): 429–30.

Cushman, John H., Jr. "After 'Silent Spring,' industry put spin on all it brewed." *New York Times*, March 26, 2001, A14.

D'Antonio, Michael. "Making a new mosquito." *Discover* 22, no. 5 (May 2001): 64–69.

Doctors Without Borders. "Malaria still kills needlessly in Africa." Press release, April 21, 2006.

Dobbs, David. "Run-AMC: the latest idea in vaccine funding won't cure AIDS and malaria." *Slate*, Dec. 29, 2005.

Dunavan, Claire Panosian. "Fighting the parasite from hell." *Discover* 26, no. 8 (August 2005): 1641–42.

Dye, Chris, and Paul Reiter. "Temperatures without fevers?" *Science* 289, no. 5485 (September 8, 2000): 1697–98.

Fedunkiw, Marianne. "Malaria films: motion pictures as a public health tool." *American Journal of Public Health* 93, no. 7 (July 2003): 1046–56.

Gladwell, Malcolm. "The mosquito killer." *New Yorker*, July 2, 2001, 42–51.

Harrison, Gordon. "Ecology: The new great chain of being." *Human Nature* 77, no. 10 (December 1968): 8–16, 60–69.

Hastings, I. M., P. G. Bray, and S. A. Ward. "A requiem for chloroquine." *Science* 298, no. 5591 (October 4, 2002): 74–75.

Howarth, William. "Turning the tide." *American Scholar* 74, no. 3 (Summer 2005): 42–52.

Kaplan, Robert D. "The coming anarchy." *Atlantic*, Feb. 1994, 44–76.

Karaim, Reed. "Not so fast with the DDT." *American Scholar* 74, no. 3 (Summer 2005): 53–59.

Marshall, Eliot. "Reinventing an ancient cure for malaria." *Science* 298, no. 5591 (October 4, 2002): 437–39.

McCarthy, F. Desmond, Holger Wolf, and Yi Wu. "Malaria and economic development: the need for a vaccine." *Current,* no. 462 (May 2004): 10–12.

Miller, Louis H., and Brian Greenwood. "Malaria—A shadow over Africa." *Science* 298, no. 5591 (October 4, 2002).

Morel, Carlos M., et. al. "The mosquito genome—A breakthrough for public health." *Science* 298, no. 5591 (October 4, 2002): 79.

Raloff, J. "The case for DDT." *Science News,* 12–14.

Rogers, David J., and Sarah E. Randolph. "The global spread of malaria in a future, warmer world." *Science* 289, no. 5485 (September 8, 2000): 1763–6.

Rosenberg, Tina. "What the world needs now is DDT." *New York Times Magazine*, April 11, 2004, 38–43.

Sachs, Jeffrey D. "Achieving the Millennium Development Goals—The case for malaria." *New England Journal of Medicine* 352, no. 2 (January 13, 2005): 115–16.

———. "A new global effort to control malaria." *Science* 298, no. 5591 (October 4, 2002): 122–24.

Shell, Ellen Ruppel. "Resurgence of a deadly disease." *Atlantic* 280, no. 2 (August 1997): 45–60.

Specter, Michael. "What money can buy." *New Yorker*, October 24, 2005, 57–71.

Stapleton, Darwin H. "Lessons of History? Anti-malarial strategies of the International Health Board and the Rockefeller Foundation from the 1920s to the era of DDT." *Public Health Reports* 119 (March–April 2004): 206–215.

Vogel, Gretchen. "An elegant but imperfect tool." *Science* 298, no. 5591 (October 4, 2002): 94–95.

——— ."In Pursuit of a Killer." Ibid., 87–89.

———. "Against All Odds, Victories from the Front Lines." *Science* 290, no. 5491 (October 20, 2000): 435–36.

Waters, A. P., et. al. "Malaria vaccines: Back to the future?" *Science* 307, no. 5709 (January 28, 2005): 528–30.

Wellems, Thomas E. "Plasmodium chloroquine resistance and the search for a replacement anti-malarial drug." *Science* 298, no. 5591 (October 4, 2002): 124–126.

Wellems, Thomas E., and Louis H. Miller. "Two worlds of malaria." *New England Journal of Medicine* 349, no. 16 (October 16, 2003): 1496–98.

ONLINE SOURCES

Bengali, Shashank. "Nurses leave, health care in Africa suffers." *Philadelphia Inquirer*, April 20, 2006. http://www.philly.com/mld/inquirer/news/nation/14382322.htm.

Briggs, Helen. "DNA clues to malaria in ancient Rome." *BBC*, Feb. 20, 2001. http://news.bbc.co.uk/1/hi/sci/tech/1180469.stm.

Bruce-Chwatt, L. J. "Chemotherapy in relation to possibilities of malaria eradication in tropical Africa." World Health Organization report WHO/Mal/175, May 21, 1956. http://whqlibdoc.who.int/malaria/WHO_Mal_175.pdf.

Clark, Katy, David Baron, Orlando de Guzman, and Clark Boyd, untitled report on malaria. *BBC World*, October 24–27, 2005. http://www.theworld.org/worldfeature/malaria/01.shtml.

Clarke, Hilary. "Nazis tried to halt Allies in Italy with malaria epidemic attack." *London Telegraph*, February 14, 2006. http://www.telegraph.co.uk/news/main.jhtml?xml=/news/2006/02/14/wnazi14.xml.

Coghlan, Andy. "New malaria vaccine raises high hopes." *New Scientist*, October 15, 2004. http://www.newscientist.com/article.ns?id=dn6537.

Gordon Covell, Paul F. Russell, and N. H. Swellengrebel. "Malaria terminology." World Health Organization monograph, 1953. http://whqlibdoc.who.int/monograph/WHO_MONO_13.pdf.

Fischer, G. "Presentation speech for the Nobel Prize in Physiology or Medicine, 1948." http://nobelprize.org/medicine/laureates/1948/press.html.

Fox, Maggie. "Incentives sought for drug companies that target poor." *Reuters*, March 7, 2006. http://www.alertnet.org/thenews/newsdesk/N07443335.htm.

Goering, Laurie. "WHO: 57 nations short of skilled health workers." *Chicago Tribune*, April 8, 2006. http://www. chicagotribune.com/news/nationworld/chi0604080144 apr08,1,5460136story?coll=chi-newsnatioworld-hed.

Gourevitch, Alexander. "Better living through chemistry." *Washington Monthly,* March 2003. http://www.washingto nmonthly.com/features/2003/0303.gourevitch.html.

Gubler, Duane J. "Resurgent vector-borne diseases as a global health problem." *Emerging Infectious Diseases*, July-September 1998. http://www.cdc.gov/ncidod/eid/ vol14no3/gubler.htm.

IRIN. "South Africa: Winning the war against malaria, so far." Februay 7, 2006 (via United Nations). http://www. irinnews.org/report.asp?ReportID=51577&Select Region=Southern_Africa&SelectCountry=SOUTH_ AFRICA.

Kalyango, Ronald. "KPI to make malaria drug." *New Vision* (Uganda), April 19, 2006. http://www.newvision. co.ug/PA/9/34/493831.

Library of Congress American Life Histories. Interviews with Mrs. Mary Bickett and Martin Cross. http://rs6.loc.gov/ wpaintro/wpahome.html.

MacArthur, Douglas. "Appendix B: Directive on malaria control." Office of Medical History, Surgeon General (online), April 18, 1943. http://history.amedd.army. mil/booksdocs/wwii/Malaria/appendixbrev.htm

Macdonald, G. "The theory of the eradication of malaria." World Health Organization report WHO/Mal/173, April 27, 1956. http://whqlibdoc.who.int/malaria/WHO_Mal_ 173.pdf.

Malakooti, M. M. K., Biomado, and G. D. Shanks. "Reemergence of epidemic malaria in the highlands of western Kenya." *Emerging Infectious Diseases* 4, no. 4. (October-December 1998). http://www.cdc.gov/ncidod/eid/vol4no4/malakooti.htm.

"Malaria threatens to become a superbug." *New Scientist*, March 15, 2006. http://www.newscientist.com/channel/health/mg18925422.900.html.

Mason, Betsy. "Scientists find way to cheaper malaria drug." *Contra Costa Times*, April 17, 2006. http://www.montereyherald.com/mld/montereyherald/living/health/14360106.htm.

McNeil, Donald G., Jr. "Malaria vaccine proves effective." *New York Times,* October 15, 2004. http://www.nytimes.com/2004/10/15/health/15malaria.html?oref=login&ex=1255579200&en=de6708254ddc9683&ei=5088&partner=rssnyt.

———. "Mosquito isn't a happy host for malaria, tests indicate." *New York Times*, April 28, 2006. http://www.nytimes.com/2006/04/28/science/28malaria.html.

Morris, Madeleine. "Drug fakes damage malaria control." BBC, November 14, 2005. http://news.bbc.co.uk/1/hi/health/4434686.stm.

Perry, Albert S. "Investigations on the mechanism of DDT resistance in certain anopheline mosquitoes." World Health Organization report WHO/Mal/244, Oct. 19, 1959. http://whqlibdoc.who.int/malaria/WHO_Mal_244.pdf.

"Resistance risk to malaria cure." BBC, January 19, 2006. http://news.bbc.co.uk/1/hi/health/4627938.stm.

Roberts, Anne. "Iron supplements aggravate illnesses in children in high malarial risk zones: study." *Earthtimes*, January 14, 2006. http://www.earthtimes.org/articles/printhistory.php?news=5007.

Roll Back Malaria. "The use of antimalarial drugs." An undated policy statement. http://www.rbm.who.int/cmc_upload/0/000/014/923/am_1.htm.

Sallares, Robert, Abigail Bouwman, and Cecilia Anderung. "The spread of malaria to Southern Europe in antiquity: new approaches to old problems." *Medical History* 48, no. 3 (July 1, 2004). http://www.pubmedcentral.nih.gov/articlerender.fcgi?artid=547919.

Shah, Sonia. "Don't blame environmentalists for malaria." *Nation*, March 31, 2006. http://www.thenation.com/doc/20060417/shah.

Snow, Jonathan. "Fighting malaria in Africa." *Online Newshour*, January 4, 2006 (with video). http://www.pbs.org/newshour/bb/africa/jan-june06/malaria_1-04.html.

———. "Killing a Killer." *Mail and Guardian Online* (South Africa), January 10, 2006. http://www.mg.co.za/articlePage.aspx?articleid=260916&area=/insight/insight__africa/.

Soren, David, and Noelle Soren. "The University of Arizona excavations at Lugnano, in Teverina, Italy." Personal Web site. http://www.coh.arizona.edu/lugnano/.

Spielman, Andrew. "Research approaches in the development of interventions against vector-borne infection." *Journal of Experimental Biology*, September 23, 2003. http://jeb.biologists.org/cgi/reprint/206/21/3727.

Thimasarn, Krongthong. "Malaria drug resistance in the Mekong River Valley." Roll Back Malaria, November 2003. w3.whothai.org/LinkFiles/Roll_Back_Malaria_Drug_Resistance_in_Mekong.pdf.

Thompson, Andrew. "Malaria and the fall of Rome." BBC, June 1, 2001. http://www.bbc.co.uk/history/ancient/romans/malaria_01.shtml.

Wells, Janet. "Malaria kills one child every 30 seconds worldwide, and Kyle Webster aims to stop it." *San Francisco Chronicle*, June 5, 2005. http://sfgate.com/cgi-bin/article.cgi?file=/c/a/2005/06/05/CMG3NCLBKA1.DTL.

World Health Organization. "Malaria." An educational booklet, 1999. http://whqlibdoc.who.int/hq/1999/WHO_CDS_CPC_ SAT_99.1.pdf.

————. "Malaria fact sheet." World Health Organization fact sheet. http://www.who.int/mediacentre/factsheets/fs094/en/.

————. "WHO calls for an immediate halt to provision of single-drug artemisinin malaria pills." Press release, January 19, 2006. http://www.who.int/mediacentre/news/releases/2006/pr02/en/index.html.

————. "The World Health Organization and malaria eradication." World Health Organization report WHO/Mal/162, Febuary 1, 1956. http://whqlibdoc.who.int/malaria/ WHO_Mal_162.pdf.

Web sites

http://www.gatesfoundation.org/topics/Pages/malaria.aspx
The short-term goal of the Bill & Melinda Gates Foundation is to significantly reduce the number of deaths from malaria by 2015; its long-term goal is to eradicate the deadly disease. Information about how the foundation plans to accomplish these goals is available on this site, along with information about research and program efforts by partner organizations.

http://www.rbm.who.int
Answers to a long list of frequently asked questions about malaria can be found on this Roll Back Malaria site.

http://www.cdc.gov/malaria/
The Centers for Disease Control and Prevention provides a one-stop site for anyone interested in the full range of details about the this mosquito-borne disease.

http://www.malariavaccine.org
The PATH Malaria Vaccine Initiative is working to accelerate the development of promising vaccines.

http://www.who.int/topics/malaria/en/
For a world view of malaria's impact, visit the Web site of the World Health Organization.

http://www.theglobalfund.org/EN/
Together HIV/AIDS, tuberculosis, and malaria kill more than 6 million people each year, and visitors to this Web site will learn what initiatives the Global Fund has put in place to control and eradicate these diseases.

Glossary

Anopheles
The genus of mosquitoes that carry malaria.

artemisinin
The active antimalaria agent in the qinghao, or sweet wormwood, plant.

artemisinin-based combination therapies (ACTs)
A new class of antimalaria medicines that mix drugs based on artemisinin with established drugs based on quinine.

chloroquine
The cheap, non-toxic synthetic drug used for decades after World War II to combat malaria around the world.

endemic
Constantly present in an area or country.

epidemic
A sharp increase in the number of cases of a disease, whether in an area where the disease exists, or in an area where it's unknown.

larva
The stage of the mosquito life cycle when it develops in water after hatching.

mefloquine
A synthetic anti-malaria drug developed in the early 1980s. Marketed in the U.S. under the brand name Larium.

Plasmodium falciparum
The deadliest of the malaria-transmitting parasites.

Plasmodium malariae
A malaria-transmitting parasite with relatively mild symptoms.

Plasmodium ovale
A rare malaria-transmitting parasite most often found in West Africa.

Plasmodium vivax
The most common and widespread malaria-transmitting parasite.

quinine
The active anti-malaria alkaloid in the bark of the *Cinchona* tree. For three hundred years, quinine was the only known treatment for malaria.

resistance
(1) The ability of a parasite to resist the effects of an anti-malaria drug; (2) the ability of a mosquito species to resist the effects of an insecticide.

sporozoite
The stage of the malaria-transmitting parasite that migrates from the mosquito to the human liver.

vector
An insect or other organism that carries a disease-causing agent and transmits it to human beings or another animal species.

Index

Alaric, 29-30

Alexander the Great, 12, 25-26, *26*

Anopheles mosquitoes, *13*, 15, 22, 38, 47, 60-61, 74-76, 80-81, 83-84, 94-95, 99-100, 102, 104, 119

Artemisinin, 106

Atabrine, 67, 69

Attila the Hun, 30, *31*

Baikie, William Balfour, 54

Beauperthuy, Louis Daniel, 57

Brazil, 83, 87, 101, 104-105

Caesar, Julius, 12, 27

Calisaya, 50-52, *50*

Candau, Marolino, 83

Carson, Rachel, 92-94, *92*

Centers for Disease Control (CDC), 77

Ceylon (Sri Lanka), 77-78, 80, 86, 95

China, 106-107

Chloroquine, 69, 71, 90, 96, 102, 106, 118-119

Cinchona, 42-44, *43*, *45*, 47-49, 51, 67

Columbus, Christopher, 33-34, *34*, 39

Cromwell, Oliver, 44, 46

Dichloro-dipheyl-trichloroethane (DDT), 71, 73, 75-84, 86-87, 91-96, 112, 114, 116, 118-119

Galen, 27-28

Gorgas, William Crawford, 61, 63-64, 72

Global Malaria Eradication Programme, 83-84

Greece, 80, 82

Hippocrates, 24

Hispaniola, 33-34

India, 87, 89, 99, 101, 114

Italy, 74-76, 87

Jamestown, 36-37, *37*

Kenya, 108

Khan, Genghis, 12

King, Albert, 57

Lariam (mefloquine), 102

Laveran, Louis Alphonse,
    57-58, *58,* 60
Ledger, Charles, 50-52
Leo I, Pope, 30, *31*

Madagascar, 11
Mamani, Manuel Incra, 50-52
Manson, Patrick, 60
Mozambique, 114, 118-119
Müller, Paul, 73, *74,* 76
Mutis, Jose Celestino, 47

Nigeria, 11

Panama, 61
Paris green, 72-74, 78
Park, Mungo, 54
Plasmodium, 16-19, *17, 59,* 67
    Falciparum, 19, 24-26,
        30, 34-35, 38, 40, 57,
        67, 83, 90, 95-96,
        106-107, 117-119
    Malariae, 19, 23-24,
    Ovale, 19, 23, 67
    Vivax, 18-19, *19,* 23, 34,
        38, 67, 84

Quinine, 43-44, 46-47, 49-50,
    52, 54-55, 63, 65-67

Rockefeller Foundation, 66,
    72, 74-76, 83
Rome, 11, 27-30, 32, 42, 44

Ross, Ronald, 55, *56,* 60-61
Russell, Paul, 83

Sardinia, 76, 80, 101
Shakespeare, William, 12, 32
Stanley, Henry, 54
Solumbrino, Agostino, 42, 44
Soper, Fred, 82-83, *82,* 87
South Africa, 114

Talbor, Robert, 47
Tanzania, 109
Tennessee River Valley,
    78-80, 101
Thailand, 10

Uganda, 116

Wilder, Laura Ingalls, 12, 64
World Health Organization
    (WHO), 82-84, 86, 89-90,
    93-95, 97, 102, 107-109

Zeidler, Othmer, 73